GO AHEAD, STOP AND PEE

RUNNING DURING PREGNANCY AND POSTPARTUM

KATE MIHEVC EDWARDS, PT, DPT, OCS
BLAIR GREEN, PT, DPT, OCS

Printed in the United States of America First Printing, 2019
ISBN 978-0-9997950-3-3

Editing by Sara Hinton
Cover design & book design by Noah Adam Paperman

Dedication

We dedicate this book to all of the incredible, strong,
passionate, and beautiful mother runners out there
that just want to run and live an active life.
You got this, girl!

Table of Contents

Acknowledgments   vii

Introduction   1

1. Our Mother Runner Stories   5

2. Running & Injury   21

Part One: Pregnancy

    3. Dispelling Pregnancy Myths   35

    4. The Pregnant Runner   41

    5. Pelvic Health   55

    6. Exercises for Pregnant Runners   65

Part Two: Postpartum

    7. Dispelling Postpartum Running Myths   91

    8. The Postpartum Runner   95

    9. Common Pelvic Floor Dysfunctions   105

    10. Musculoskeletal Injuries in Postpartum Runners 119

    11. The Postpartum Runner Is Different   135

    12. Preparing to Run   147

    13. Time to Run   237

    14. Go Out There and Kill the Hills   257

About the Authors   261

References   265

Acknowledgments

This project has been more work than we could have imagined—and completely worth it. We are so grateful and humbled by all of the support we have received along the way. This book would not have been possible if it were not for our supportive families and husbands, who listened to us day in and day out as we were excited, frustrated, tired, and excited again about this book.

Thank you to Jackie Merritt for being our model for our long and tiring photo shoot. Not only was she a fantastic model, but she has been a great supporter of this project from the moment we told her about it. She is the beautiful pregnant runner we have on our cover and the model in the "Prepare to Run" exercise section of this book.

Thank you so much to Coach Carl Leivers for contributing to the two running programs that we have included in this book. He is an incredible running coach and a great resource for runners all over the country. He is also a husband and father of two beautiful little girls, and he understands that chaos and the beautiful imperfection of life can get in the way of running, but that it doesn't have to ruin your running goals.

Thank you to Samantha Taylor for letting us use her incredible image on our cover. Thank you to Tracy Sher and Pelvic Guru for allowing us to use some of her images throughout the book. Tracy is an athlete, physical therapist, and mom who has dedicated her career to educating others about the power of physical therapy for women, and ensuring that women can find health care providers in their geographical areas. We are so grateful.

Introduction

We are moms. We have both been on the receiving end of the health care system. We have seen and felt the lack of support women receive during pregnancy and postpartum around exercise and running. We believe that there needs to be better education surrounding exercise for women during pregnancy and postpartum. We strongly support exercising during pregnancy and postpartum to maintain a healthy lifestyle, provided there are no contraindications.

This book has been a labor of love for both of us. We have been excited, nervous, frustrated, and simply done with writing at various points during this process. It has been said that writing a book is like giving birth—we disagree. Giving birth to a human is much more difficult! However, there are so many similarities and emotions in both processes.

The first version of this book was very clinical. Then we read it and realized that for it to truly mean anything to another woman, we had to be more open and authentic about our experiences. We have truly tried to be vulnerable and let you see a glimpse of what our lives look like as both moms and runners.

However, as physical therapists that treat other moms, we wanted to make sure we gave you the best possible information. That is why this book is a series of stories and experiences intertwined with science. We are nerds. We love science. But we want you to actually enjoy this book as you learn! So, bear with us as we take you through the journey of running during pregnancy and postpartum. We hope you love it and learn something on every page.

When I became pregnant, I knew I wanted to continue running as long as possible, and that I would eventually return to running after I had my son. When I started to research what I could and could not do, I didn't find a lot of information, and I didn't know where to look. This left me scared and confused. Then, when I went to see my first OB/GYN, she immediately told me I would not be able to continue running. The short story is that I fired her immediately. The longer story appears in a few pages. I quickly found a physician who was more supportive of my plans and goals. She was up to date on the most current evidence, which supports staying active throughout pregnancy; she also understood the research, and that running during pregnancy would not harm me or my baby.

My story is not all that different from those of other women. When I became pregnant, I was concerned and even scared that I would do something wrong that would hurt my baby. One of the biggest pregnancy myths is that you should not run because it is "bad for the baby." Later in this book, we will discuss all of the research that supports running and exercise during pregnancy and dispel some common myths.

Running is an attractive exercise option for moms. It is much easier to lace up your shoes and run out of the door than it is to go to a gym. For me, running was a gift; it allowed me a few minutes of alone time, as well as some much-needed freedom, by taking my son with me on the run. One of the many benefits of maintaining an active lifestyle postpartum is that women who run while breastfeeding have a significantly lower incidence of postpartum depression[1].

I know that if I hadn't been able to get outside nearly every day, I would have had a far more difficult time transitioning into motherhood.

We recognize the lack of information and resources for women who want to run during pregnancy, who want to return to running after the baby is born, or who start their running journey postpartum. Most women have no idea where to start, what to expect, how their bodies should feel, and what is and isn't normal. By addressing these issues and educating others and ourselves about how our bodies change during pregnancy and the months following childbirth, we can significantly reduce the stigma and fear around running—as well as the potential for both injury and other long-term consequences.

In 2018, the American College of Obstetricians and Gynecologists (ACOG) released a committee statement redefining the "fourth trimester" of pregnancy, stating postpartum women should receive continued care and guidance following the birth of their child.

This is a significant leap forward for women in the United States; it finally recognizes that the physical and psychological changes of pregnancy continue well after childbirth. Yay! It is about time.

When I was pregnant, I used my physical therapist brain to poll all of my running friends, look through research, and ask my doctors. I found that there was a serious lack of information available about running through pregnancy. After my son was born, I was lucky enough to work with Dr. Blair Green PT, DPT, CSCS, and the co-author of this book, and she gave me some great guidelines about returning to running. Between my expertise in running and her expertise in women's health, we figured it out. Since then, we have collaborated extensively to treat female runners during pregnancy and postpartum.

Our guess is that you are reading this book because either you treat female runners or you are a runner who is pregnant or postpartum. Unfortunately, we did not have this resource for ourselves, but I am so excited to share it with you!

You will see that our treatment approach is evidence based and clinically relevant. Our goal for this book is to educate health care professionals and women who just want to run (or keep running). We hope it empowers you to help yourself or your clients through this incredible chapter of life. Now, let's begin with our stories.

Happy running.

With love,
Kate

Our Mother Runner Stories

Kate's Running Story

I love running. I love everything about it. How it makes me feel physically, emotionally, and psychologically. I love the sound of my feet as they hit the pavement, the wind in my face, and the smell of laundry when I run past someone's house. Running has always been my exercise, my sanity, my freedom, and my community. Prior to getting pregnant, I ran all of the time, as much as I possibly could. I did 5Ks, 10Ks, half marathons, marathons, and relay races that lasted twenty-four hours, and I even began dipping my toes into the world of triathlon. In fact, I was training for a half Ironman distance triathlon when I found out I was pregnant. Since it was going to be my first Ironman, I did not do it, but I continued to stay very active.

Every woman feels differently about her pregnancy. I knew I wanted a family but never felt ready—ever. The day I realized I was pregnant was terrifying for me. One morning I woke up and tasted metal in my mouth. I thought it was my vitamins, so I threw them all away. Another morning, I felt sick to my stomach, and I assumed I had eaten something bad. Then, a few days later, I went out for a friend's birthday and had a few drinks. The next morning, I was so sick I could barely get off of the couch, and I hadn't had much to drink. Then I noticed my boobs felt huge. I remember my friends saying that beer doesn't make your boobs get bigger overnight. I was convinced it did.

Over the course of the next several days, I locked myself in the bathroom, and I took more than ten home pregnancy tests. They were all positive. However, I somehow convinced myself I couldn't possibly be pregnant. I was freaking out. After I took the very last test I had in my possession, and it was positive yet again, I called my best friend. I tried to get her to agree with me. I tried to get her to tell me that I couldn't possibly be pregnant.

After much gentle coaxing, she talked some sense into me and convinced me to unlock the bathroom door, go downstairs, and tell my husband. After a lot of silence, it sunk in. I finally realized I was pregnant. I slowly unlocked the door, walked downstairs, and told my husband. I still remember exactly where he was standing in the kitchen, fiddling with the radio on the counter. I remember the look of pure happiness on his face and how he was immediately thrilled. He was beaming, and all I wanted to do was throw all of the pregnancy tests at him.

I know a lot of women have a difficult time getting pregnant, and I questioned even writing the truth about how I felt at first.

But I promised to be authentic, so here it is. It wasn't that I was ungrateful or angry that I was pregnant. It was the opposite. I was excited and happy, but I had always been so terrified of change. Having a baby was the biggest life change I could imagine, and a change I wasn't sure I was ready for. I loved my life. I loved training for races. I loved running for as long and as far as I wanted without having to come home for any reason. I loved the freedom. It took me a little while, but I got excited, too, in between the daily nausea, throwing up, and extreme exhaustion.

Like many couples, my husband and I decided not to tell anyone for several weeks, but when I went to go for a bike ride and my bike tire popped, I sat on the ground crying uncontrollably. Not the quiet, pretty tears: the ugly, red-faced sobbing ones that I was fairly sure my neighbors could hear. It didn't take long for my training partner, a mother of two, to recognize the signs and figure it out! The secret was out of the bag, and I was relieved. Now I had someone to answer all of the questions that were swirling inside my brain. Why do I feel crazy? Am I supposed to feel this sick? How do I stop throwing up? Can I keep training?

I was determined to continue running and exercising throughout my pregnancy, but I met resistance along the way. The first person who objected was my OB/GYN, who I briefly mentioned in the introduction. At my first appointment, I asked her for tips for how to stay active during pregnancy, since I had never been pregnant before. I assumed she would be the best resource, but I was so wrong. Before I had even finished talking about how I wanted to keep running, she began lecturing me that I shouldn't be running at all, and that I needed to be more careful now that I was pregnant. I only heard part of the lecture, because after her statement, "You shouldn't keep running," I heard nothing she said the rest of the visit. I was so angry. I was educated, and I had read the available research, yet she treated me as if I were a child.

Prior to pregnancy, I was emotional, but as the hormones started to change, I was a very special kind of emotional. Sometimes, I felt as if I was watching the evil version of myself, but there was nothing I could do to stop it. Other times, like when my bike tire popped, I cried and cried as if someone had told me my dog died. So, I wasn't sure if I was overreacting or being too emotional when she told me I couldn't run. At my second appointment, I brought my husband for backup. Thank God. I was *not* overreacting. *She* was wrong. When we left the second appointment, we fired her. Luckily, I found an amazing doctor after that who supported my wishes.

I was sick for six of the nine months of my pregnancy. The first three months, I was nauseous and throwing up every day, all day. Sometimes I would be treating patients and would have to run out of the room, apologizing as I barely made it to the bathroom. Then I had a blissful second trimester, followed by another three months of being sick. I tried everything to stop getting sick, like eating only crackers, consuming large amounts of ginger, wearing the little bracelets with pressure points, and taking medication.

The only thing that helped me was running. The more I ran, the less sick I got. So, I continued to run as much as possible. I ran before work and after work, and every weekend I ran eight to ten miles on Saturday, and a few on Sunday. I continued to run regularly and listened to my body along the way. I also did pregnancy yoga every week, rode my bike, and lifted some light weights. I ran a half marathon while six months pregnant and loved it. Secretly, I loved passing people, only to hear them say, "Wow, did you see her? She's pregnant!" as I ran by. I participated in a few other races and always wore my "Running for two" T-shirt, flaunting my big baby belly!

Every single day was different. Some days I woke up and had the energy to go two miles; other days I went eight. Some days I didn't go at all, and instead, I lay on my bed passed out and drooling because I was so tired. As my belly got bigger, I had to create running routes that had several bathroom stops along the way. I ended up getting a Gabrialla support belt for my belly to help hold it up as I ran. It helped me a lot for most of my pregnancy. My belly wasn't the only problem, though; my breasts also were huge. I was amazed at how large they got. It seemed like every few weeks I was getting larger sports bras to support them. Finally, I found a bra called "the Ta Ta Tamer," and all of my problems were solved.

I also found that I got overheated much more easily. I must tell you I don't like the heat. I live in Atlanta, and every April through October, I complain about it. Not a little complaining; *a lot* of complaining. So much complaining that my friends have offered to buy me an ice vest and a fan to carry around so that they might see me during the summer months. Being pregnant only made me despise the heat more. My house is always cold, but when I was pregnant, it was an icebox, and my lovely husband had to wear wool socks and a jacket to bed. I had to stay very hydrated, and I often wore short sleeves, even in winter, to prevent overheating with exercise.

The further along I got, the slower I ran. In the last month of my pregnancy, I thought I was running, but I probably looked like I was waddling or walking, or something in between. I ran until somewhere between 36 and 38 weeks, and then I gave in and started walking.

From the moment I stopped running, I wanted my pregnancy to be finished. I wanted to have my baby. I started walking up and down hills, doing squats in my backyard, being more intimate with my husband, eating eggplant Parmesan, and trying anything I read online or in magazines about how to have my baby sooner.

None of it worked. He came when he was ready, at 41 weeks. I listened to my marathon-long run mix all of the way to the hospital, and it helped me focus. I imagined that I was running a race.

My birth story is long and hilarious, but I will spare you the details since this is a book about running, not birth. I was lucky to have had an un-medicated, uncomplicated birth. My birth went so well I thought I would start running immediately. To my surprise, my body didn't agree.

In many countries around the world, women are pampered after giving birth, spending months resting, during which their primary job is to heal. Not in America. We beat ourselves up for not getting back to our pre-baby body in a month. We constantly judge ourselves and pick ourselves apart from the moment the baby is born. I know I did.

I had this very American idea and timeline in my head about what my body was supposed to do, and when. The day after I had my son, I remember looking down at my flabby, empty baby belly in disgust. I didn't tell myself I was amazing for pushing this nearly nine-pound child out of my vagina, with no medication, the day before. Instead, I started judging myself. I hope you treat yourself with much more love and respect than I did. If I knew then what I know now, I would have said something like, "Wow body, you are amazing!"

I was sorer, moved more slowly, and was much more tired than I had anticipated. Like many women before me, I thought I would bounce back after a few days, but I didn't. I had some lingering back pain from my back labor, as well as hip pain for a few weeks. I would notice that if I sat cross-legged or moved too quickly, my hip would catch. I was bleeding heavily (no one tells you about this part!), my vagina hurt, and my nipples were cracked, bleeding, and in pain from breastfeeding. Not to mention I was exhausted from not sleeping, emotionally drained, and completely in love all at once.

I started my road back to running with walking every day. My son was born in April, so it was beautiful outside. I started walking around the block and eventually began walking several miles. I did Pilates every week, and he came with me. As he slept, I did not sleep. Instead of taking that age-old advice, I wrote a course called "The Endurance Athlete". I prepared lectures, read running research, and dreamed about my next race. I also started my basic breathing exercises and some strength exercises that I often gave my own patients postpartum. Eight weeks after having my son, I saw Blair for a pelvic floor checkup. I had always told my postpartum runners to do this, but clearly, I had never experienced it.

Even though I was in the physical therapy business, I was still nervous. Everything went fine, though. Blair watched me move, observed my mobility and strength, and eventually looked at my pelvic floor. She was able to identify that the right side of my pelvic floor was tighter than the left (my right hip was the hip that was hurting), but overall, everything looked okay. The small amount of tearing I had was healing, and she said I could start to do a little running. I saw her for a total of four visits to work on my posture, breathing, and the tightness in my pelvic floor. I learned so much and felt so much better for having gone to see her.

I started to do a combination of walking and running at first. Then, I was so happy to be running that I ignored everything I knew and just went for it. I started ramping up my mileage too quickly, however. I was pushing a stroller (with a car seat in it), plus I was exhausted and breastfeeding, and probably could have worked on my strength longer.

Within a month, I had a stress fracture in my left foot and was put in a boot. I was forced to stop running for another month. Talk about angry. I had just got my freedom back, and it was gone again! I hate to say it, but yes, even physical therapists make stupid mistakes! My love of running got the best of me.

Once my stress fracture was healed, I was much smarter. I listened to my body when I was tired and I walked/ran slowly, building up my base to run. When I began running consistently again, I was so very grateful. I was able to run a few short races and eventually a couple of half marathons. This is where I wish my story ended. I would like to say I am now running marathons and back to doing triathlons without any trouble, but that's not what happened. But what happened next was not because I had a baby.

Around the time of my son's first birthday, I began to notice I was more tired than most new moms. I was falling asleep at seven in the evening, and I was having a difficult time staying awake all day. I had to stop during my runs and catch my breath, and my heart felt like it was beating so hard with every step I took. It also felt like it was skipping beats. I thought it was because I had a young baby and that I was tired, doing too much. That I was just out of shape and breastfeeding. But that wasn't it. I found out I have a rare, genetic heart disease called arrhythmogenic right ventricular cardiomyopathy (ARVC), and that forced me to stop running altogether.

Again, I won't go into the whole story, because this book is about running during pregnancy and postpartum. How it is possible, worth it, and completely amazing to continue doing what you love during this season of your life! I also wrote a whole book, *Racing Heart: A Journey of Love, Loss and Perseverance*, about my journey of being diagnosed with ARVC and dealing with the loss of running, if you want to learn more about it.

These days, I am no longer running, but I am still very involved with the running community. My practice, Precision Performance & Physical Therapy, is a niche clinic focusing on the treatment of runners and triathletes. I write books and articles and speak about running all over the United States. I still love running, and want you and your patients to be able to continue to run during pregnancy, and then get back to running postpartum, with as much information and ease as possible! I hope you enjoy this book.

Blair's Running Story

I wish I could say I was a marathon runner or a super sprinter. My earliest running memory was third or fourth grade, when we had to run the 600-yard timed test in PE. I was one of the last to finish. I would dread conditioning for cheerleading because it was June and we had to run a mile around the track. How could four laps really be so far? I was always active in sports, so I never thought to run for exercise until college. I had stopped cheering and playing softball and needed a way to stay in shape. Duke University had two campuses separated by a mile-and-a-half-long road. I forced myself to run back and forth, and somehow started to enjoy it. In physical therapy school, I was in Philadelphia, and there was a beautiful path by the river that I would occasionally run. My best friend in school also ran marathons, and even today on runs I hear her in my head: "You have to kill the hills…kill the hills!"

It wasn't until I moved to Atlanta that I began to run races. It was convenient, inexpensive, and social. I ran my first AJC Peachtree Road Race (an annual 10K on the Fourth of July) in 2000, and ran it every year until my second pregnancy in 2007. I skipped that summer because I just was not comfortable running in the heat, but I picked right back up again the following year. I loved the idea of setting a goal, training, and accomplishing the goal. I did *not* love running in the heat or humidity, and even worse was the cold of winter. Having goals and commitments made it easy to continue running. However, it was also easy to stop during pregnancy because my body just did not feel good from pounding the pavement. I chose to cycle and use the elliptical trainer instead, and continued to work out through both my pregnancies.

About thirty weeks into my first pregnancy, I began to notice my blood pressure creeping up. I checked in with my OB/GYN and was diagnosed with pre-eclampsia. This is also known as pregnancy-induced hypertension, and can be a medical emergency. If I did not stop not only exercising—but also most physical activity—I was at risk for liver and kidney problems, as well as seizures.

I was immediately placed on bed rest. For a woman who was starting a new PT practice, teaching Pilates, and focused on staying active with friends through exercise, this was devastating. I didn't know how to sit still (I still don't know how!).

Until that day I was diagnosed with pre-eclampsia, I had my first delivery all planned out. I read all of the books and wrote down my birth plan. I signed up for childbirth classes and a hospital tour. I planned everything, so why would it not be that way for my labor and delivery?

Pre-eclampsia meant my actual birth story would look very different. I was on bed rest first at home, and then in the hospital. I underwent an emergency C-section three weeks later, and my son spent the first month of his life in the NICU. I was deconditioned and exhausted, pumping around the clock, and spending every free moment at the hospital.

Exercise was not in the cards—at least not at first. I started doing small exercises at home instead, like pelvic clocks and bridges, as well as low-intensity abdominal work. When I was finally cleared to exercise, I took my son for walks in the stroller and eventually started running. He was too small for my new running stroller, though, so I could only go if my husband was home to watch the baby. For a woman who had been exercising nearly seven days a week up until point, this was a big change, and took a lot of adjustment.

I slowly regained my strength and stamina, and a year later, I completed my first half marathon (another goal to check off of my list). That same day, I also sustained my first running injury—a right hamstring strain. I took a little time off and went back to training when I could. After all, the AJC Peachtree Road Race was only a few months away. It may have been a blessing in disguise, but I soon became pregnant again, and stopped running. I learned from the first time around that, for me, running and pregnancy just didn't mix. My hip was still not at 100 percent, and it was easy to make that decision.

Here's where the story gets a little crazy, however. I stopped running in July 2007. My hip pain went away eventually, and I could exercise through my entire pregnancy. It was uncomplicated, and I did not deal with blood pressure issues at all. My daughter was born in February 2008 via C-section. I was able to recover from surgery quickly, and started on the same postnatal regimen of exercises I had done after my first delivery. I went back to my OB/GYN for my six-week postnatal check, and he gave me a green light to run. I did not assess my strength, posture, balance, or running form. I did not try to ease back in with a run/walk program. I simply went to the gym and hopped on the treadmill.

BAM! Hip pain. Right then. Immediately.

What was going on?

I was certain that my injury had healed months ago, even though I continued to battle hip pain off and on for many years. After struggling through pain but not being willing to stop exercising, I finally did all of the "things" I should have done in the first place. I had my running form assessed, switched shoes (minimalist shoes were the thing at the time), got custom orthotics, ditched the orthotics, went to PT, did Pilates, and started cross-training.

I did so much during that time that I don't remember what actually worked. Something did, though, because I no longer experienced hip pain while running, but I think that was just a coincidence, not the result of something I actually did to get rid of it. I also continued to run. The entire time! I had goals to meet: more half marathons, mom boot camp classes, group runs.

It's amazing how the PT has so much trouble being the patient. We know everything not to do, but in my case, I was not listening to my own body. Running was an easy and quick way to get my exercise in. Juggling two kids, work, and other commitments was not easy! My daughter did not love running in the stroller, so that was even more limiting.

At one point, my husband and I were taking a group fitness class. I would go to the early session, and he would meet me with the kids in between the classes, when he'd join the second class. Then I would drive the kids home. We got creative so we could both get our runs in. In the meantime, I was still growing my practice, and that took time. The recovery from baby number two was significantly longer than the first time around. Looking back, I am certain I could have done many things differently that would have both sped up my recovery and also helped me deal with the hip injury.

My love/hate relationship with running continues today. I have figured out that running thirteen miles is enough for me. No marathons are in my future. I keep a steady 9:30-10:00-minute-per-mile pace on longer runs, and that is pretty consistent. When I have a friend to run with, a commitment to meet, or a goal to crush, I run more.

When it's up to me, I find something else to do. I still find an occasional race to keep myself committed and motivated. I also keep my kids active, and we have made exercise a priority in our family lifestyle. This mindset makes it easy to walk out of the door and run on a Sunday morning. My kids know this is a regular part of our lives. They don't question it. They don't think I'm choosing running over them. They know that a healthy mom is a healthy family. Sometimes (though very rarely), they join me. On those days, I don't run as far or as long.

What I've learned through all of this is how to be flexible. Sometimes the best-laid plans don't always come to be, and we need to show respect and care for our bodies in pregnancy as we make our way back to our active lifestyles. Remember: It's important to respect what your body is trying to tell you and not beat yourself up if you are not where you want to be at any given point in time.

What I've also realized is that I am pretty lucky. I am a physical therapist who works with women. I know a lot about how to return to exercise postpartum. Most women do not have the correct information—or any information. They feel lost and unsupported in their efforts to stay active or to become more active after they've had children. They seem resigned to a life of continual exhaustion, leaking, pelvic pressure, not being able to wear two-piece bathing suits, and so much more. What's worse is that society seems to have normalized this: T-shirts discussing our extreme fatigue or inability to do jumping jacks; blogs and memes and social media that glorifies all of the things moms deal with that they don't have to.

After practicing physical therapy for nearly 20 years, I decided to re-dedicate my career to being there for moms. My practice, Catalyst Physical Therapy, was created to give women a place to feel loved and supported, and to give them the tools and empowerment to use their bodies however they see fit. It is my wish that this book gives you a little hope that you can return to a sport you love, and show you that there are people out there who want to help you reach this goal.

WHAT YOU NEED TO KNOW

» Injury happens to nearly all runners.

» Training error is almost always why we get injured.

» Injury is multifactorial and sometimes unpredictable. It can occur because you stepped in a pothole, you are too stressed out, you are doing too much, too soon, or you have a dysfunctional movement pattern.

» Male and female runners are quite different.

2

Running & Injury

Injury is one of the worst things that can happen to a runner. Having to sit on the sidelines as you watch your friends, training partners, and even random people on the street run by you is excruciating. Even if you love your friends, sometimes hearing them talk about their splits, their last wonderful run, or their most recent race experience can put you over the edge. We understand. We have both been there on the sidelines, on one or more occasions.

This chapter covers everything you need to know about running injuries. It is based on the research that is available and our clinical backgrounds. It is not specific to the pregnant or postpartum runner, but will serve as a launch point for delving deeper into the specifics concerning these populations. This chapter will also give you an in-depth understanding of the differences between male and female runners, why injury occurs, and what the causes of injury usually are. Be warned: it is technical and full of research!

Today, there are more than thirty-five million runners in the United States, and more than half of them are women. According to the most recent data from Running USA's National Runners Survey, a majority of runners run to stay healthy, stay in shape, relieve stress, have fun and socialize, and be a part of a group. Many women begin running after having a baby to get back in shape, to get out of the house, or to meet other moms in their situation. Running postpartum and being part of a community can also even prevent the onset of postpartum depression.[1] It creates a much-needed support system of other women who share similar experiences, or sometimes it simply provides a mental break. Running can help women maintain their identities as people with real names, goals, and lives outside of being a mom.

Despite the many benefits of running, injury often gets in the way. Each year, 19 to 92 percent of runners are injured. This wide range of incidents exists because there is significant variation in the definitions of running injuries, and there are inconsistencies within studies. Many factors affect the statistics regarding running injuries, such as differing populations of runners, varying follow-up periods, and much more[2,3].

Despite these inconsistencies, it is clear that running injuries are a common obstacle for both runners and health care practitioners alike. According to the most recent National Running Survey, 75 percent of runners have had an injury in the last twelve months; 50 percent of these people had to take more than four days off from training, and only 27 percent sought medical attention. Much needs to be done to help reduce the injury rates of runners and improve the care and education they receive about a physical therapist's role in healing running injuries[4].

In our practice, we have found that more often than not, our clients are relieved when they finally come in to see us. They are relieved because they didn't know they could get better faster with care than without. They didn't know they could be taught the means to prevent many injuries from happening in the future.

The foot hits the ground somewhere between 800 and 1500 times during a mile run, with forces anywhere from 1.5 to five times your body weight[5,6]. The slower a person runs, the more steps taken per mile. Why does this matter, you might ask? It matters because the more steps a runner takes per mile, the more opportunities for injury, and the more load for the body to manage over time[6]. Increased body weight, quickly changing body posture, center of mass, and many other physiological factors that face women during pregnancy or postpartum may put women at high risk for injury.

The point of training is to cause enough stress on the body and its tissues to improve strength and bone density, and to promote positive tissue remodeling. However, too much stress, with inadequate recovery time, leads to a breakdown of tissues[7]. In other words, if training loads increase too quickly or too much, the musculoskeletal system can become overloaded.

This includes increasing daily or weekly mileage, or not incorporating rest time into training plans. The continuous, low-grade forces placed on the body during running begin to break down tissue faster than it can repair itself. In the clinic, runners often say things like, "This injury came out of nowhere!" But when we look back at their training volume, training intensity, and the various stresses in their life, we are often able to see that they were setting themselves up for injury for days, weeks, months, or even years without realizing it.

A majority of running injuries are due to overuse. Overuse injuries are caused by the combination of stress and repeated microtrauma in the bones, muscles, joints, ligaments, and tendons. Overuse injuries may occur without a single, identifiable causative event[7]. This is what makes overuse injuries so frustrating. You may not even realize you are overloading yourself, and then you become injured. Stress is stress, however, and it will be discussed further in Chapter 7.

In contrast, too much rest and not enough stress at the tissue level can cause the tissue to become weaker over time, and resuming training at the previous load applied becomes far too much for the body to tolerate[7]. An example of this is when a runner takes an extended amount of time off during pregnancy, and then after the baby is born, begins training exactly as she was training pre-pregnancy. The runner trains with the same amount of mileage, intensity, or duration, without taking into consideration the time off or the changes the body has undergone throughout the pregnancy and delivery. The runner may become injured because the tissues are weaker, and therefore can become overloaded sooner than they previously did. Both too much load and not enough load over time can cause overuse injuries in runners.

Amount of load is not the only factor in overuse injuries. The rate and direction at which a joint is loaded can impact tissue breakdown. This is important because it illustrates that biomechanical and structural factors, such as arch type, hip adduction angle, knee valgus, increased stride length, excessive eversion, pelvic drop, and excessive pronation can also predispose runners to injury[7-10].

There are also kinetic factors that predispose the runner to injury, including but not limited to rate of impact loading, magnitude of propulsive forces, and magnitude of impact loading[7]. Gait analysis is an effective way to determine if a runner is predisposed to overuse injuries because of biomechanical and structural factors. In layperson's terms, the way the body accepts load when the foot hits the ground can be a factor in injury. There are various changes that occur in pregnancy and postpartum, such as the arch and the pelvis widening, that need to be considered for the prevention and the rehabilitation of injuries.

Overuse injuries occur slowly, and often it is difficult to determine when or how the injury occurred[11]. Common overuse injuries that occur in all populations of runners include patellofemoral pain syndrome, iliotibial band syndrome, posterior thigh pain (hamstring/back of the leg), medial tibial stress syndrome, stress fractures, lower back pain, Achilles tendinopathy, ankle sprains, and plantar fasciosis[5,7].

There is some debate as to whether there is a difference in injury based on sex. Some literature has found that there is not a significant difference between male and female runners, but more recent evidence has suggested that sex is a predictor for injury[12,13]. Van de Worp et al. found that the factors that increased the risk of running-related injuries in women but perhaps not men were as follows: older age, previous participation in non-axial sports (e.g. cycling, swimming, etc.), participating in a marathon in the last year, running on concrete, engaging in a longer weekly running distance (48–63.8 km), and training in the same pair of running shoes for four to six months[3].

Risk factors for running injuries are generally categorized as intrinsic (age, sex, menstrual cycle, fitness levels, alignment, body structure, and biomechanics), or extrinsic (shoes, orthotics, training, training surface, or equipment)[5,10]. Many of the extrinsic risk factors in running injury are similar in men and women. Previous injury and training errors are the most common causes of injury in runners.

Training errors often mean that the runner did too much, too soon, with too much intensity—whether the runner realized it or not. Clinically, training errors are incredibly common. We have found that collaborating with a knowledgeable running coach is invaluable, especially for runners that are injury prone. Novice runners, those that have run fewer than three years, are also at a higher risk for injury. Other extrinsic factors that contribute to injury are taking any extended amount of time off and then returning to running and/or to a higher mileage than the body can tolerate[3,4,13,14].

More recently, a greater emphasis has been placed on the role of health and lifestyle factors as a risk for developing running injuries. These include smoking, alcohol, stress, and previous injuries, amongst other things. There are many health and lifestyle factors the postpartum athlete faces that are of significant consideration when it comes to injuries. New moms are often exhausted from lack of sleep, possible anemia or thyroid issues, recovery from childbirth, and simply adjusting to a "new normal." They have different nutritional needs, especially if they are breastfeeding, and there is an increased amount of emotional stress as they negotiate their new life. Ten to 20 percent of postpartum women suffer from postpartum depression, and exercise has been shown to improve this condition[15].

Although physical therapists are not trained to treat postpartum depression directly, many who work with this group have the ability to properly identify warning signs among mothers, and are able to refer them to an appropriate mental health provider. Physical therapists also provide an outlet for safe movement and exercise, and can support moms as they work through the challenges of postpartum depression. Although many of the stressors mentioned above that occur postpartum are risk factors that precipitate injury, exercise, including running, is important to mental health and overall wellness.

DIFFERENCES BETWEEN MALE AND FEMALE RUNNERS

To further understand running during pregnancy and postpartum, we first need to comprehend how female runners are different from male runners. The literature shows that women have different physiological, biomechanical, and psychological issues than men.

Female sex hormones can influence the physiological impact of exercise and performance. For instance, where a woman is in her menstrual cycle can affect her energy levels, thermoregulation, and blood flow[16,17]. During the first one to seven days of the menstrual cycle, estrogen levels are the lowest, and then during days eight through 11, estrogen surges to induce ovulation.

Both estrogen and progesterone increase slowly until approximately days 19-21, when they peak and begin to decline. The literature has demonstrated that the higher the estrogen in the body, the lower the body's core temperature, and then improved heat dissipation occurs[16].

Additionally, during the luteal phase of the menstrual cycle (approximately days 11 through 25), higher progesterone levels increase the core body temperature threshold for both sweating and cutaneous vasodilatation. These differences are more significant when the runner is untrained. As a female runner becomes more aerobically trained, there are fewer fluctuations in sex hormones affecting sweating and thermoregulation[17,18]. In fact, the onset of sweating is closer to that of her male counterpart the more trained she becomes[18]. It may be necessary to adapt the training schedule based on where a woman is in her menstrual cycle, especially for women who have just begun training.

Both men and women have the hormones testosterone, estrogen, and androstenedione, but the ratios of production between the sexes are different. In general, women have one-seventh the amount of testosterone that men do. These differences are why women tend to have a higher percentage of body fat (22-26 percent) than men (13-16 percent), and demonstrate less muscle mass. Increased levels of estrogen in women are responsible for the higher percentage of fat in female runners[10,19]. Testosterone and androstenedione create leaner body mass, larger cross-sectional areas of muscle, and increased strength in men, compared to women[10,16]. In other words, women have smaller muscles, less strength, and higher percentages of body fat compared to men. These differences in body composition play a role in how the body tolerates and responds to training.

Despite the fact that women have less strength and smaller muscles than men, during exercise, their muscles tend to fatigue more slowly and recover more quickly than men's. This is believed to be true because women's muscles generate less force, which improves blood flow and oxygen to the muscles. Women also have different neural factors and differences in skeletal muscle fiber type[16]. So next time you see a man sprint by you, remember that in the longer run, you might just pass him!

Men and women also have physiological differences in their cardiovascular systems that impact their cardiac output, oxygen transport, blood pressure, and VO2 max[10,16]. Women have smaller body frames, lungs, and thoraxes. This results in smaller heart size and heart volume, which ultimately results in a lower stroke volume (amount of blood circulated with each heartbeat). They also have 30 percent less cardiac output (cardiac output = stroke volume x heart rate) than men because of their lower stroke volumes.

Moreover, women have fewer red blood cells and 15-20 percent less hemoglobin than men, which leads to a lower oxygen-carrying capacity and oxygen uptake[16]. The decreased blood volume and decreased hemoglobin contribute to a VO2 max that is typically five to 15 percent lower than men, with comparable training status[16] and 15-25 percent lower after controlling for differences in body weight and percentage of body fat[10]. In other words, the blood cell makeup of women compared to men affects their ability to become aerobically trained. All of these factors have been cited as reasons why there are substantial differences in the performance of male and female runners.

Biomechanical differences between men and women also affect how they move. Some of the differences in women compared to men include increased knee valgus, increased hip internal rotation, increased hip adduction angles, and a wider pelvis. The wider pelvis of female runners is the basis for lower extremity differences in women, as it leads to increased femoral anteversion, genu valgum, and hip adduction angle[10]. Increased hip adduction angle has been cited as a major factor in lower extremity injury[5,9,20-22]. This is one example of how altered biomechanics affect the way the bones and joints are loaded with running, and potentially place female runners at a greater risk for lower extremity injuries.

Additionally, women tend to have decreased muscle strength compared to men, particularly in the hip abductor and external rotator muscles[10,20]. These muscles control the stability of the pelvis and leg, especially while standing on one leg. They also demonstrate decreased response time and shock absorption at the knee and ankle joints, making it more difficult to control the lower extremity through dynamic motions, such as running and lateral movements. These are some of the reasons that differences are seen in the way women run, jump, and land[10]. In terms of running, women also take more steps per minute than men do at equal speeds[1,6]. As previously stated, an increase in steps taken means that there is increased load through the lower extremities, which may increase the risk of an overuse injury.

Beyond physical differences, the most recent National Runners Survey from Running USA found that men and women often have different reasons for running. Although both men and women run for health, fitness, and weight loss, as well as to be competitive, women tend to run for social benefit more frequently than men.

Women typically use running as a means to spend time with friends, get out of the house, build a social support network, have fun, and be a part of a community. The loss of running because of injury can therefore be more devastating to women from a psychosocial perspective.

Men and women have differences physiologically, biomechanically, and psychosocially when running that impact the rate and types of injuries they sustain and how they are affected by these injuries. The differences between male and female runners become exponentially more complicated when pregnancy is introduced into the equation. The remainder of this book will focus more specifically on pregnant runners and postpartum runners.

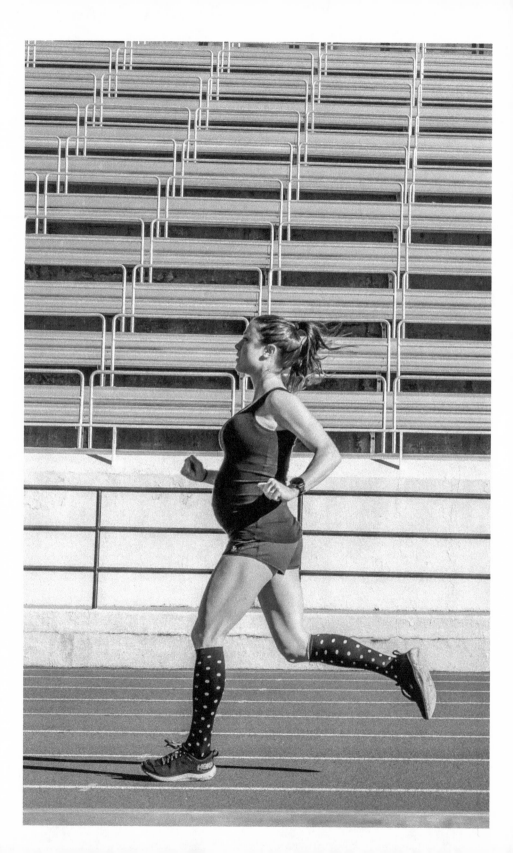

Part One: Pregnancy

3

Dispelling Pregnancy Myths

I n our clinics, we always have to re-educate our patients about information they read online or that their friends or training partners may have told them. Learning from other women and their experiences can be valuable. But, much like the game of telephone, information passed along from woman to woman often gets muddled along the way. We asked members of our tribes to help us put together this list of common myths and misconceptions, and then we went ahead and gave you the truth—nothing but the truth.

Myth 1:

Women shouldn't run while they are pregnant.

Truth:

In general, this is not true, unless you have a medical issue and have been told you cannot run because of it. If you have been running prior to pregnancy, then most women are fine to continue running. You may have to modify how much and the intensity based on how you feel.

Myth 2:

Running during pregnancy will put too much pressure on my bladder muscles and cause future leakage.

Truth:

Unfortunately, some women do have urinary incontinence when running while pregnant and postpartum, but this is not normal. If it happens, you should seek out a women's health specialist. Many women run their entire pregnancy without any urinary incontinence. Moreover, the presence of urinary incontinence during pregnancy does not mean it will continue following delivery or cause leakage in future pregnancies. There are many reasons why a woman may experience urinary incontinence while pregnant, including when running while pregnant. A women's health specialist should be able to determine the cause and figure out the best course of treatment.

Myth 3:

Running while pregnant increases stress on the baby (i.e.: it might be shaken, overheated, or deprived of oxygen), and is not a good idea.

Truth:

Research has found that for healthy women, exercising during pregnancy is not associated with preterm birth. Exercising during pregnancy can actually decrease risk for cesarean delivery, preeclampsia, and gestational diabetes, and it can also decrease both musculoskeletal pain and birth weight (to a healthy range).

Myth 4:

Running during pregnancy will cause a diastasis recti abdominis, or separation in the abdominal wall.

Truth:

Diastasis recti occurs in up to two-thirds of women during pregnancy. The separation is due to lengthening muscles and fascia and is a normal change during pregnancy. Running does not increase the chances of having a separation, or the severity of the separation.

Myth 5:

Running will increase my heart rate too much and hurt my baby.

Truth:

In the past, doctors have recommended that women keep their heart rate in a certain range while exercising during pregnancy. This is a challenge because heart rates at rest and with exercise are based on your level of fitness and exercise intensity. Not every woman has the same heart rate while running. An acceptable guideline is to run at a comfortable pace at which you can carry on a conversation.

Myth 6:

I shouldn't do abdominal exercises when I'm pregnant.

Truth:

There is no harm in doing abdominal exercises during pregnancy. As pregnancy progresses, the size of your abdomen and the stretch of your muscles will make exercise more difficult. It is okay to modify positions and move in smaller ranges of motion to minimize straining and reduce the risk of injury. Continuing modified abdominal exercises is not harmful to mom or baby.

Myth 7:

If you weren't exercising before you were pregnant, don't start now.

Truth:

Exercise has been shown to be beneficial during pregnancy (see Myth 3). The American College of Obstetrics and Gynecology (ACOG) recommends that women exercise during most days of their pregnancy. Certain types of exercise may have more risk and should not be started during pregnancy, however. These include activities that involve a high level of skill and balance. Moderate cardiovascular exercise, weight training, and even yoga and Pilates are acceptable forms of exercise during pregnancy.

Myth 8:

Running will send you into labor.

Truth:

Labor is triggered by hormones. This is a coordinated event where the uterus, fetus, and brain are all communicating with each other. Running does not affect these communication pathways and will not trigger labor. Severe cramping, contractions, and bleeding, however, are signs of overexertion, or perhaps a more significant medical problem. If you experience any of these symptoms while running, stop immediately and contact your doctor.

Myth 9:

Your body needs to rest and be a calm place for the baby.

Truth:

For all of the reasons previously stated, exercise is beneficial for mom as well as the growing baby. There is a difference between staying active and participating in regular exercise and performing high-risk activities, such as diving or sports with a high-fall risk. Most of the studies on trauma to the fetus are based off of data from motor vehicle accidents. Running and moderate exercise do not deliver this type of trauma or force to the growing fetus. Again, ACOG recommends regular exercise as part of a maternal health plan.

WHAT YOU NEED TO KNOW:

» It is smart to run with a friend, or at the very least, a phone, just in case.

» Stay hydrated: You often need more water than you might think.

» As your belly and breasts become larger, get support so that you can be as comfortable as possible (we have some suggestions for support at the end of this chapter).

» Run at a pace that allows you to hold a conversation with someone.

» Don't beat yourself up as you get slower or if you aren't up to running as much as you used to. Everyone is different, so don't compare what you are able to do and comfortable with to what others have done.

4

The Pregnant Runner

Running during pregnancy is more common than ever. There is a whole new industry of running shirts with statements such as: "Running for two," "Yes, my doctor says it's okay to run," and "No, I did not swallow a pumpkin!" Research has proven that for most women, running during pregnancy is a good thing.

What you need to understand as a pregnant runner or health care provider is that the body undergoes tremendous physical change during pregnancy.

Underestimating what is happening in the body can cause frustration when running times get progressively slower, or when typical runs of three to five miles seem much more difficult. Understanding the changes the body is undergoing will allow pregnant women to run more confidently. It will also help health care providers treat their clients more effectively.

While some changes occur rapidly and early on in pregnancy, others develop gradually. Each trimester (13 weeks) of pregnancy is characterized by its own set of physiological changes. Some of these changes are visible, such as weight gain and postural adaptations. Others, including cardiovascular and hormonal changes, are not as obvious, but are equally significant. There is overwhelming support for exercise during pregnancy[23]; however, understanding your body's changes will help you understand what is a normal response to exercise and what may require more attention.

WEIGHT GAIN

The Institute of Medicine updated its recommendation for weight gain in pregnancy in 2009. It recommends a weight gain of 25-35 pounds for singleton pregnancies.

This may vary from person to person. Factors include pre-pregnancy weight, activity level, and fluid retention. It is recommended that women who are underweight gain up to 40 pounds during pregnancy, while those who are overweight not gain more than 15 pounds. Pregnancy weight may include the weight of the fetus, placenta, breast tissue, fat stores, and fluid. Research shows that continuing to exercise throughout pregnancy does not seem to affect gestational weight gain, dispelling a myth that exercise may harm the growth of the baby. Also, remember that it is not appropriate to use exercise during pregnancy as a means to minimize or prevent weight gain[24,25].

BONES, JOINTS, AND LIGAMENTS

The skeletal and ligamentous structures in the body support the growing fetus. They also help prepare the body for childbirth by becoming more "lax." As the baby grows, the mother's posture begins to change. The rib cage may become flared, and the natural arch in the spine, known as lordosis, may increase. Increasing lordosis may cause the pelvis to tilt anteriorly and tighten the hip flexor muscles[26]. The thoracic spine may also become more rounded as breast size increases. Some women develop more of a swayback posture, with the hips and pelvis anterior to the shoulders, and a posterior pelvic tilt[27]. Hormones, such as relaxin and progesterone, affect all of the body's connective tissue[28]. In the bony skeleton, the pelvis widens, primarily at the joint in the front, the pubic symphysis. Joints may feel "looser" or easier to stretch than they felt prior to pregnancy. The arches of the feet may flatten.

Another change in the joints is a reduction in synovial fluid. Synovial fluid is the lubrication for the joints (like oil in an engine). It is important to recognize this change because it may take longer to warm up joints while exercising[29].

MUSCLES

The muscular system adapts to the changing bony framework of the skeleton. With changes in posture, the muscles may lengthen or shorten. Moreover, laxity in the ligaments may place more demand on the muscular system to provide support with movement[27].

Muscles that typically become tight include lumbar paraspinals, psoas, iliacus, hip flexors, adductors (inner thigh), and pectoralis muscles (chest).

Muscles that typically become lengthened include abdominals, hamstrings, glutes, and posterior shoulder muscles.

A common occurrence in pregnancy is a stretching of the fascia (connective tissue) in the abdominal wall at the linea alba (midline).

This is known as diastasis recti abdominis (DRA), and affects up to two-thirds of all pregnancies[30]. Tissue laxity, coupled with a stretching abdomen, causes this to occur. It is not an emergency, and with appropriate attention and modifications, there is no reason a woman cannot exercise with DRA. Exercise modifications for DRA will be discussed later.

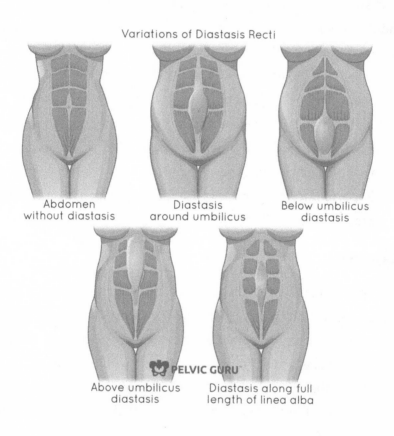

Diastasis Recti Abdominis, courtesy of Pelvic Guru

CARDIOVASCULAR

Cardiovascular changes begin in the first trimester. Like the ligaments, the blood vessels also become lax. Blood pressure initially decreases. This is known as "underfill." The biggest symptom of underfill is dizziness with position changes. During the second trimester, blood volume begins to increase and can increase up to 50 percent by the end of the second trimester. Blood pressure returns to normal postpartum.

Varicose veins are a common occurrence in pregnancy. It is common to see varicose veins in the legs, as well as in the vulva[31]. The risk of varicose veins increases in pregnancy because of laxity in the blood vessels. Compression garments may help minimize the varicosities and improve circulation.

In the first trimester, there is also an increased demand for oxygen. Heart rate increases in response to this demand[31]. If you monitor your heart rate while running, you may find that it is higher than normal, or increasing rapidly as you begin to exercise. It may be necessary to slow your pace, for the warm-up or for the entire run, especially as pregnancy advances.

In the third trimester, blood pressure may begin to rise. It is important to monitor it as pregnancy advances, as hypertension (blood pressure greater than 140/90) is a sign of a medical emergency known as pre-eclampsia. Other signs of pre-eclampsia, or pregnancy-induced hypertension, include swelling in the legs and ankles, headaches, right-sided upper abdominal pain, blurred vision, and rapid weight gain (over one to two days).

One phenomenon to consider with exercise is supine hypotension. This occurs around week 20 of pregnancy and can continue through delivery. It happens when the pregnant woman lies on her back. The weight of the fetus can compress the inferior vena cava, which is the main vein that returns blood to the heart. The result is a drop in blood pressure, which can leave the woman feeling dizzy or lightheaded, and in some extreme cases, can even cause the woman to pass out[27]. The important thing to know about supine hypotension is that when it occurs, it does not harm the baby at all. Still, there is some evidence that at full term, lying supine may impede blood flow to the fetus[31]. It is also completely preventable by limiting the amount of time that the pregnant woman spends on her back while exercising. Many exercises and stretches can be modified to standing, side lying, or sitting to prevent supine hypotension.

PULMONARY

The demand for oxygen increases in pregnancy, with half of all oxygen inhaled going to the uterus. In addition, the shape of the diaphragm may change, due to its attachment to the rib cage, as well as the growing fetus leaving less room for this muscle to descend on inhalation. Respiratory rate may increase to accommodate these changes; however, the pulmonary system does a good job of adapting to maximize oxygen absorption with each breath[31]. Increasing warm-up time and lowering running pace can help minimize the risk of shortness of breath as pregnancy progresses.

RENAL

A common side effect of pregnancy is increased urine output. While the size of the uterus may affect the frequency of urination, the amount of urine being excreted also increases. This is important to remember, as runners may notice having to stop more frequently for bathroom breaks while out on a run. Using the restroom "just in case" or holding urine too long may both lead to future risk of pelvic floor dysfunction, such as urinary incontinence. However, limiting fluid intake before or during runs is not advised, as this puts the woman at risk for dehydration. There is a greater need for fluids in general during pregnancy[31], and even more so with running, due to the loss of fluid through sweating.

ENDOCRINE

Hormones, including estrogen and progesterone, rise during pregnancy to help support the growing fetus, as well as the placenta[28]. Estrogen and progesterone are produced in the adrenals, but during pregnancy, are also produced by the placenta. These hormones, in addition to relaxin, prepare the body for childbirth by increasing laxity in connective tissues. The mother's body also begins to prepare for lactation, an event stimulated by estrogen.

BIOMECHANICAL

During pregnancy, women demonstrate decreased step length and stride length, increased base of support, and increased double limb support time (time spent on both legs) during walking and running[24,26,32]. These physiological changes continue for at least eight to 16 weeks postpartum[32,33].

BENEFITS OF EXERCISE DURING PREGNANCY

Physiological changes help prepare the body for pregnancy and delivery. It is equally important to prepare the mind for the changes that will occur during pregnancy, and for childbirth and motherhood in general. Multiple studies show that exercising for at least 30 minutes on most days of the week at a moderate intensity will produce many positive physical and psychological effects, including:

- Increased energy
- Improved mood
- Better sleep
- Decreased incidence of depression
- Increased social connections
- Reduced risk of gestational diabetes
- Lower weight gain during pregnancy
- Easier loss of post-pregnancy weight

Evidence shows that exercise during pregnancy helps preserve or slightly increase a woman's aerobic fitness without risk to the mother or to the developing fetus[24]. By six to eight weeks postpartum, the uterus and vagina have returned to their pre-pregnancy size[27]. It is around this time that women usually return to the OB/GYN for their postpartum check-up. If there are no complications from the delivery, they are typically given a green light to slowly resume their previous level of activity.

RECOMMENDATIONS

In the past, many doctors were hesitant to recommend exercise to pregnant women because little was known about the effects on mom and baby. However, research in the last 10 years overwhelmingly supports exercise during pregnancy. In 2017, the American College of Obstetrics and Gynecology (ACOG) updated its guidelines, not only supporting, but also recommending up to

150 minutes of exercise per week, at a moderate intensity, during pregnancy.

The meaning of "moderate intensity" varies from woman to woman. Those who train year-round and who have built up endurance may be able to tolerate faster speeds and longer runs compared to women who do not run as often or at a competitive level. Regardless of level of fitness or running experience, it is important to include at least a 10-minute warm-up before advancing to your typical running pace. Due to the physiological changes of pregnancy, the body needs time to respond to the demands of running through a longer warm-up[29].

Pregnancy weight gain will increase the amount of force that moves through the body due to the high-impact nature of running[32]. With each step, the ground reaction force, the amount of force that travels from the ground up through the body, increases as well. Maintaining strength in the hips, low back, and core can help support the increased load. It may be necessary to decrease the running pace or distance to limit excessive load on joints as pregnancy progresses.

Pregnancy is not a time to try something new, like significantly increasing distance or running a marathon for the first time. How much is too much? One conventional method to gauge the correct exercise intensity is known as the "talk test." While running, your heart rate will rise, but you should still be able to carry on a conversation with a friend.

In addition, hydration is important. Drinking water before, during, and after exercise is recommended. In general, hydration needs are greater during pregnancy, and this is especially important with exercise, when body temperature rises and fluid is lost. Just remember, you may need to plan a running route that has more bathroom stops than normal!

Other signs that intensity is too high include:

- Chest pain
- Headache
- Shortness of breath
- Lightheaded or dizzy feeling
- Calf pain
- Muscle weakness
- Bleeding from the vagina
- Leaking of fluid from the vagina
- Uterine contractions

If any of the above symptoms occur while running, stop immediately and call your doctor.

SUPPORT

Pregnancy is a dynamic process, and changes can occur rapidly. Musculoskeletal aches and pains are common. Running may exacerbate this discomfort; however, many women continue to run even with pain or discomfort. Changes in biomechanics, posture, center of gravity, joint laxity, ligamentous laxity, and weight may all contribute to difficulty with continuing to run as pregnancy progresses.

Companies have capitalized on the large population of pregnant runners by creating braces and other types of external support devices to help women continue running throughout pregnancy. We recommend consulting with a physical therapist before using any of these supportive products. Most of them are not harmful, but some may be more beneficial than others.

The most common type of support is a lumbar and/or pelvic belt or brace. These typically contain elastic and have a Velcro closure. They are designed to support the spine as pregnancy advances. A disadvantage to this type of support is that long-term use may discourage use of your own muscles to support your spine through reliance on the brace. However, for people who run longer distances, they may be helpful.

Another alternative is support shorts, which may also offer compression. Standard shorts work well early in pregnancy, but may not be comfortable with a growing belly due to the compression. Some brands make a type of compression short with a cutout for the belly. These shorts may also aid in circulation, which can be compromised due to laxity of blood vessels, and help with varicosities in the legs and pelvic region. As a general rule, any compression garment should not restrict blood flow, especially to the lower abdomen and pelvic region.

Proper footwear for exercise during pregnancy is essential. Women may need greater arch support and cushioning, as ligamentous laxity will affect the feet. In addition to new, supportive shoes, orthotic inserts can also provide additional support and cushioning. As with postural supports, we recommend consulting with a physical therapist before purchasing any shoes and/or orthotic inserts. This will ensure proper type and fit, minimizing the risk of injury.

PRECAUTIONS/CONTRAINDICATIONS

As stated, exercise is recommended throughout pregnancy. It enhances mood, moderates the physical changes that can occur with pregnancy, and may aid with postpartum recovery. Certain conditions may require special clearance from a physician before you start to exercise, however, or may require you to modify or discontinue your exercise routine. The list below outlines the known precautions and contraindications. If you are experiencing any of these symptoms or conditions, please consult with your obstetrician before starting or continuing to exercise[34].

- Heart disease
- Lung disease
- Cervical insufficiency/cerclage
- Pregnant with multiples
- Risk of preterm labor
- Placenta previa after week 26
- Rupture of membranes
- Pre-eclampsia or high blood pressure
- Severe anemia

Being mindful of the changes that occur during pregnancy and the warning signs that you are over-exerting is key to being able to continue to run safely throughout pregnancy. It is okay to slow down your pace, run less frequently, or take more breaks to walk. Do what is comfortable for you. With the proper modifications, you should be able to find your groove out on the road, even if it's a little different than what you were doing before you became pregnant. Be smart, listen to your body, and stop if something does not seem right. Otherwise, enjoy the time you have to breathe, think, and prepare, or just lose yourself in thoughts that have nothing to do with baby or motherhood.

WHAT YOU NEED TO KNOW:

» The pelvic floor muscles are always working at a low level.

» The pelvic floor works in coordination with the diaphragm, lower back, and abdominals.

» The pelvic floor can be injured even if you have a cesarean delivery.

» The first three months after you give birth are considered the fourth trimester, and moms need continued care during this time.

» We believe all women should receive postnatal screening for musculoskeletal health.

5

Pelvic Health

L et's jump right into one of the least talked about but probably most important things to consider both during pregnancy and after having a baby: the health and function of the pelvic floor muscles (PFM). Yes, the pelvic floor is made up of muscles! Like every other part of the body, pregnancy can and does affect the function of the PFM. This region of the body undergoes significant change, including stretching, extra work, possible tearing, and ultimately recovery through the pregnancy and postpartum period.

WHAT IS THE PELVIC FLOOR?

The PFM are the group of muscles that attach between the pubic bone and tailbones[35]. They create a hammock-like structure and function in many ways, including:

- Support of the urinary and genital organs
- Control of both bowel and bladder
- Sexual function, such as arousal and orgasm
- Stability and postural control—they are the inferior part of the "core"

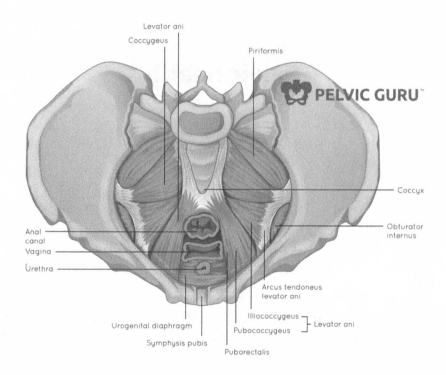

The Pelvic Floor, courtesy of Pelvic Guru

The PFM are always working at a low level. The muscle fibers are 70 percent Type 1, which makes them primarily endurance muscles. The other 30 percent are Type 2 muscle fibers, which are involved in strength and power. The PFM help maintain posture, allow the body to respond to movement, and are involved in the control of what is known as intra-abdominal pressure (IAP). The

PFM work in coordination with the abdominals, diaphragm, and lower back muscles to control the rise in IAP[36].

During running, IAP rises each time the foot hits the ground. In other words, the PFM are working harder with running to control impact forces and to maintain alignment and posture. This is why re-learning to breathe properly and control the PFM has such a profound effect on injury prevention in runners.

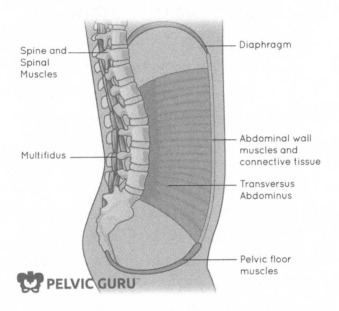

Spine and Spinal Muscles

Diaphragm

Multifidus

Abdominal wall muscles and connective tissue

Transversus Abdominus

Pelvic floor muscles

PELVIC GURU

The Diaphragm, courtesy of Pelvic Guru

The PFM lengthen and stretch during pregnancy. Changing posture, a growing abdomen, and the need to prepare for childbirth all contribute to the lengthening of the muscles. The weight of pregnancy alone is enough to increase the load on the PFM.

Increased length + Increased load = Greater demand on muscles

Similar to other muscles, such as the hamstrings or quadriceps, if a muscle is overloaded, it becomes susceptible to injury. Pregnancy is a time when muscles are working at a greater capacity. The body adapts throughout pregnancy so that the muscles do not become overloaded. However, the risk of pelvic floor dysfunction rises with pregnancy and childbirth due to the increased demands placed on these muscles[37].

THE PELVIC FLOOR AND CHILDBIRTH

Compare labor and delivery to a marathon; it is hours of lengthening and activity of the PFM, and physical activity for the entire body. The PFM are at risk of further strain, and there is a potential for injury, including stretching and tearing of the muscles, and excessive stretch to the nerves in the pelvis. Tears to the PFM occur in one-third of vaginal deliveries[38]. The pudendal nerve, which innervates many structures in the pelvis, can stretch up to 15 percent more than its regular length[39]. Many women experience tears in the perineum, which may require sutures. Following delivery, the PFM, nerves, and soft tissue structures benefit from a period of relative rest. The PFM require recovery time, much like other muscles after an injury, and a slow return to pre-pregnancy levels of activity. In fact, the number one risk factor for pelvic organ prolapse later in life is childbirth.

THE PELVIC FLOOR AND CESAREAN SECTION

Undergoing a cesarean section may eliminate childbirth damage to the pelvis and perineum, but it does not eliminate the risk of injury to the PFM. A great deal of the overload to the muscles occurs during pregnancy itself, and is not dependent on the method of delivery. In addition, some women may do some pushing before requiring a cesarean delivery. A cesarean section is major surgery, and incisions require time to heal. This will be discussed further in Chapter 8. Ongoing scar management can help speed recovery. The abdominal incision in a cesarean section goes through the many layers of abdominal fascia. Starting abdominal exercises or running too soon after delivery may impact how the tissue heals. Adhesions may form, and at a minimum, the tissue needs time to repair itself and strengthen before placing loads on it through running and high-level exercise.

Recall the relationship between the PFM, abdominal muscles, low back, and diaphragm. These muscle groups work together as a team. If one muscle group is injured or not working appropriately, the system cannot function efficiently.

Regardless of mode of delivery, the PFM are at risk of injury, and the likelihood of pelvic floor dysfunction following delivery may increase with a return to running prematurely. We know that getting back to running as soon as possible is important. However, how you approach running can impact your risk for injury, both immediately and several years down the road. Think of recovery as training for a marathon. Don't set yourself up for failure early on.

THE FOURTH TRIMESTER

The concept of a "fourth trimester" reflects the ongoing need for care for the mom after the baby is born. Many cultures emphasize postnatal care, providing physical and psychological support for mothers during the immediate postnatal weeks. Unfortunately, this is not the standard practice in the United States. Typical medical care following childbirth is a postnatal follow-up visit with the OB/

GYN or midwife, occurring approximately six weeks after delivery. The examination involves checking to see if the uterus has returned to its pre-pregnancy size, that there are no signs of infection from sutures or tearing, and that the tissue is healing. It is also a time to address any concerns the woman may have.

Some providers will screen for postpartum depression, which, according to the CDC, occurs in one out of nine women giving birth. The provider may or may not instruct the woman to perform Kegel exercises. In fact, a 2011 study surveying over 200 women about childbirth and pelvic health showed that only 58 percent of women interviewed were familiar with Kegel exercises[40]. Moreover, many women were not aware that performing pelvic floor muscle retraining could help prevent bowel and bladder impairments following childbirth. These statistics demonstrate a lack of education about postnatal women on the part of their health care providers.

The good news is that the approach to postnatal care in the United States may be changing in the near future. ACOG released a committee opinion in May 2018 recognizing the fourth trimester and calling for improved standards of postnatal care for women[34]. It is the hope of many that this recognition by ACOG will set a new standard for maternal health, and that women's physical, emotional, and social needs following childbirth will be addressed in a more comprehensive manner.

Physical therapists who are trained in pelvic health already have the tools to assess postnatal function of the pelvic floor muscles. It is our belief that all women should receive an evaluation by a pelvic health physical therapist prior to returning to running and any other form of exercise. Pelvic floor dysfunction, including pelvic organ prolapse and urinary/fecal incontinence, can be prevented with early intervention, such as learning how to properly contract and relax the pelvic floor muscles, how to correctly build strength and endurance of these muscles, and how to integrate pelvic floor muscle function with the abdominals, low back muscles, glutes, and the entire body[40]. Seeing a pelvic health physical therapist is not a substitute for the postnatal exam performed by the OB/GYN or midwife; it is an additional assessment focused on tissue mobility, posture, and muscle function as they relate to everyday activities, including childcare, job demands, housework, and recreational activity, such as running.

The postnatal physical therapy evaluation should occur between four and six weeks after childbirth, for both vaginal and cesarean deliveries. This gives the muscles and soft tissue time to recover from childbirth, but still allows for early intervention to regain basic motor control of the pelvic floor and abdominal muscles. Once the physician or midwife clears the woman to return to exercise, she can then slowly ramp up her program, following the recommendations given by the physical therapist.

In most cases, only one or two visits to the physical therapist is necessary. Typically, the physical therapist will prescribe specific exercises and recommendations for how to return to more intense physical activity, such as running. Some women may require eight to 10 visits for more detailed exercise instruction, manual therapy, and monitoring of return to activity, and a few will need significant intervention due to severe impairments, such as incontinence, muscle weakness, or pain.

The need for a prescription from a physician to attend physical therapy is a misconception. In many states, a woman can receive a physical therapy evaluation without a referral. Please refer to Chapter 12 for resources to find a physical therapist who can perform a postnatal evaluation.

While we believe that all women should receive a postnatal screening for musculoskeletal health, not everyone will have immediate access to a physical therapist immediately following childbirth. The exercises outlined later in this book are designed as guidelines to follow when returning to exercise.

While every woman should work at her own pace, certain scenarios may call for further evaluation by a physical therapist. If you answer "yes" to at least one of the following questions, pelvic floor dysfunction may be present. The likelihood of pelvic floor dysfunction increases with each "yes." If these symptoms persist for more than three to six months following delivery, and/ or you have tried the exercises suggested in this book without success, we recommend you contact a physical therapist for a more comprehensive examination.

PELVIC HEALTH PT CHECKLIST

Answer YES or NO to the following questions:

Do you leak urine at any time, even just a few drops?

Do you struggle with constipation?

Do you avoid certain types of exercise because of leaking urine, or do you wear a pad "just in case" while you exercise?

Do you feel an extreme urge to urinate or defecate, like you won't make it to the bathroom on time?

Do you have pain in the pelvic region with sexual intercourse?

Do you have hip pain that is not resolved with rest or any exercises you have tried?

Do you have low back pain that is not resolved with rest or any exercise you have tried?

Are you pregnant or have you given birth, either vaginally or via cesarean section?

Do you experience pressure in the lower abdomen or pelvis?

Do you feel like something is "falling out" of your vagina or rectum?

Have you undergone pelvic or abdominal surgery but continue to have pain or symptoms?

Do you feel like pelvic pain, pressure, or leaking urine/feces is keeping you from performing all of the activities you would like?

6

Exercises for Pregnant Runners

P regnancy is not the time to push your body to reach new strength, running limits, or PRs. It is a time to improve and maintain the strength and mobility you already have, and enjoy running/moving your body as much as possible.

As noted in the previous chapters, the goal of exercise during pregnancy is to remain active. If you had an exercise program prior to pregnancy, continue doing it. It should be a combination of stability, mobility, and cardiovascular exercises. If you experience any of the complications or precautions previously stated, stop exercising until you see your doctor. The following exercises are meant to be an adjunct to what you are already doing. They are the exercises we think will benefit you the most during pregnancy. We selected them because we think they will set you up to be in a better place to return to running postpartum.

FOUNDATIONAL EXERCISES

Practice these exercises as often as you can, ideally daily. Building a strong foundation you will decrease your risk for injuries later on.

1. Diaphragmatic Breathing

Breathing is the hallmark of any good muscle training program. Women often substitute breath holding for optimal core muscle activation. The reality is that the diaphragm works with the abdominals and pelvic floor muscles to coordinate core control. Having non-optimal breathing strategies, such as breath holding and/or bearing down with effort, can exacerbate pelvic floor dysfunction and diastasis recti. Good diaphragm function actually helps the pelvic floor contract properly. Ideally, the diaphragm, abdominals, and pelvic floor muscles should all work together.

Breathing is also a great way to facilitate improvement in pelvic floor muscle activation at all stages of pregnancy, and while the PFM are recovering from childbirth.

If you are in the first trimester, you can start by lying down on your back, with your knees bent in a comfortable position. If you are in the second or third trimester, modify the exercise by lying propped up on a wedge or on your side, or by sitting or standing. Find the position where your pelvis is not completely arched nor tucked. This is called neutral pelvis. For a full description of neutral pelvis, see Chapter 11. It can be more challenging to find neutral pelvis during pregnancy because of all of the postural changes that occur, especially later in pregnancy. Finding neutral pelvis is important, however, as it allows us to breathe well in any position we may encounter as part of normal life function.

Take a deep breath in. As you inhale, focus on feeling your ribs expand and your belly and chest rise. At the same time, your pelvic floor muscles should be lengthening and relaxing. Your diaphragm is a dome, and when it contracts, it flattens. As that occurs, the pelvic floor also moves inferiorly, but it is lengthening (this action of the pelvic floor is opposite of what the diaphragm does). Coordinated movement of your ribs, chest, and abdomen is a sign of a good diaphragm contraction.

As you exhale, the opposite should occur: your diaphragm rises, your pelvic floor and abdominal muscles contract, and your ribs, belly, and chest move downward and inward.

Continuing this breathing pattern will not only help the pelvic floor muscles contract, but will also help them relax. For optimal muscle function, a full range of motion is important. In addition, breathing through the diaphragm helps bring oxygen to the muscles, and soft tissue and helps overall relaxation.

Practice breathing 10-15 full breaths.

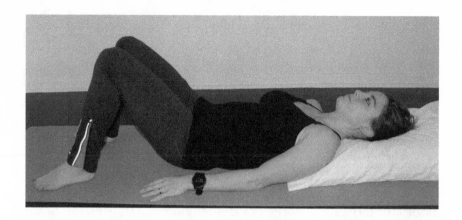

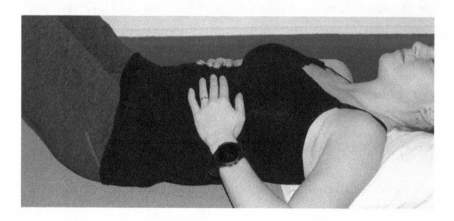

Diaphragmatic Breathing (continued)

2. Pelvic Floor Retraining (Kegel Exercises)

Pelvic floor dysfunction is associated with postnatal problems, such as urinary and fecal incontinence, as well as pelvic organ prolapse. Retraining the pelvic floor muscles has been shown to be an effective way to prevent, improve, and eliminate these symptoms. Remember, this exercise is about building the foundation and helping you maintain your PFM strength and function as the muscles stretch through pregnancy. As mentioned previously, more pressure is placed on the PFM during pregnancy because of the growing fetus and changes in posture and ligament laxity. Maintaining PFM strength is helpful as pregnancy advances to counteract some of these changes.

Perform this exercise on your back in the early stages of pregnancy, or propped up on a wedge on your side with your knees bent as your pregnancy progresses. A good way to progress the exercise is to then try to perform the exercise on all fours or while sitting on a chair, in the car, or even on an exercise ball.

Perform one diaphragmatic breath (see exercise #1 above). Begin a second breath with an inhale. As you exhale, imagine a kidney bean at the opening of your vagina.

Gently squeeze and lift the kidney bean. Continue to breathe as you hold the contraction for up to 10 seconds. Relax completely before repeating.

If you cannot hold for 10 seconds, hold as long as you can for 10 repetitions. Work your way up to a 10-second hold. If this cue does not work for you, imagine you are trying to stop yourself from urinating. Lift the pelvic floor muscles up and in as you exhale to stop the flow of urine.

Continue to breathe as you hold the contraction. Be aware of your hips, abdominals, and back. Keep them relaxed: avoid tensing or tucking your glutes, pelvis, or inner thighs, and avoid holding your breath.

Goal: 10-12 repetitions, holding each for 10 seconds.

Note: Do not perform this exercise while you are going to the bathroom.

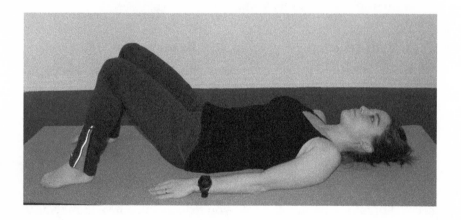

MOBILITY EXERCISES

Mobility is an important pillar of good functional movement patterns. All runners will benefit from improved spinal mobility. Ideally mobility exercises are performed daily or at the very least days you are exercising or running.

1. Cat/Cow

This exercise is good for general mobility in the neck, spine, and pelvis. Exercising in the all-fours position will help take pressure off of the lower back as the abdomen expands in pregnancy. Weight bearing through the arms will also help maintain strength in the shoulders. This exercise is not an extreme stretch. Try to move comfortably through your range of motion, and do not stretch deeply into the end of your range.

Begin by positioning yourself on your hands and knees. Line up your shoulders over your hands, and your hips over your knees. Your spine should be positioned in a neutral position (not excessively arched or curved). Watch that you are not tucking your pelvis under.

Take a preparatory breath and activate the pelvic floor muscles on the exhale. On the next breath, inhale to prepare. As you exhale, tuck your chin, letting your head and neck drop. Round your back so it arches like a rainbow. Try to get your head and pelvis as close as possible.

Inhale as you lift your tailbone, letting your stomach sink and your lower back arch. Lift your head and chest simultaneously.

Repeat 10 times.

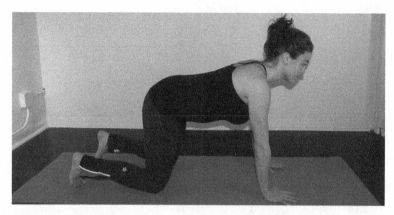

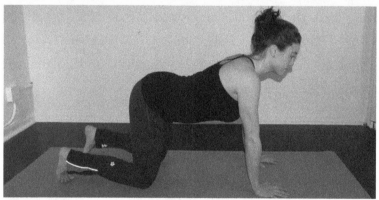

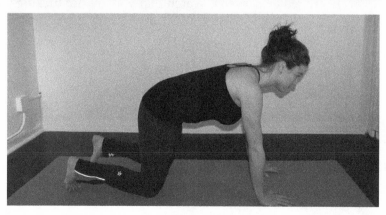

2. Thread the Needle

Like the cat/cow, this exercise provides all of the benefits of working in an all-fours position. It also adds the element of trunk rotation, specifically in the thoracic, or mid-back region, which often becomes tight from growing breasts and changes in posture.

Begin by positioning yourself on your hands and knees. Line up your shoulders over your hands and your hips over your knees. Your spine should be positioned in a neutral position (not excessively arched or curved). Watch that you are not tucking your pelvis under.

Take a preparatory breath and activate the pelvic floor muscles on the exhale. On the next breath, inhale to prepare. Exhale and slide your right arm down and under your body, reaching for your left shoulder. Your right palm should be facing up. As you move, allow your spine to rotate and stretch through the right side. Try to keep your left elbow straight.

Once you reach the end of your range, hold the position for three to five seconds and *inhale* as you lift your hand off the floor.

Exhale, and return to the start position.

Repeat 10 times on each side.

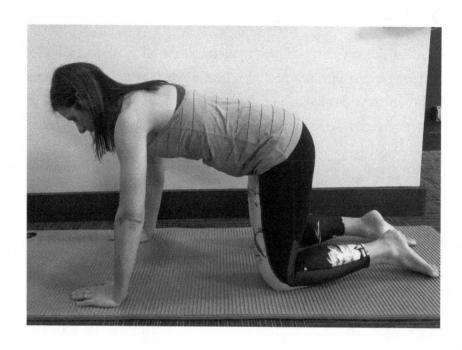

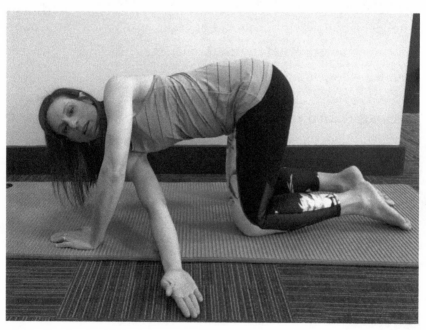

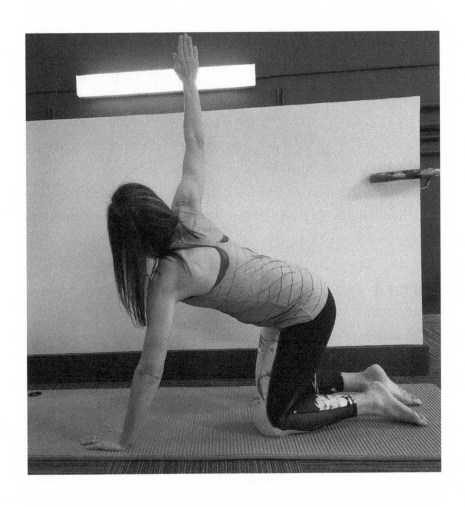

STABILITY EXERCISES

Perform these exercises every other day or at least 4 days a week.

1. Intrinsic Foot Strength

Foot strength is often overlooked because its contribution to running is misunderstood. The arch of the foot has been described as "the core of the foot." When the arch collapses under the weight of the body, there is a risk for increased pronation, internal rotation of the leg, knee valgus, and hip drop. As described in previous chapters, pronation, internal rotation, knee valgus, and hip drop have been correlated with various lower-extremity running injuries.

The foot is the first part of the body to touch the ground when we stand, walk, or run. During pregnancy, the foot gets wider and larger to support the weight above. When a runner has a weak foot, balance and single-leg strength may be sacrificed.

Therefore, building intrinsic foot strength may improve our single-leg strength and control. Running is essentially a single-leg sport. At any given moment in the gait cycle, the runner has one foot on the ground in stance phase, while the other leg moves through the swing phase.

Begin these exercises sitting in a chair. As they become easier, progress to standing, and eventually to standing on one leg while performing them.

Toe yoga:

Begin by sitting in a chair. Lift and spread your toes up and as high as you can without lifting the ball of your foot. All of your toes should spread.

Once you can do this, attempt to only lift the big toe.

Relax your toes and repeat 10-12 times, holding for five seconds each time.

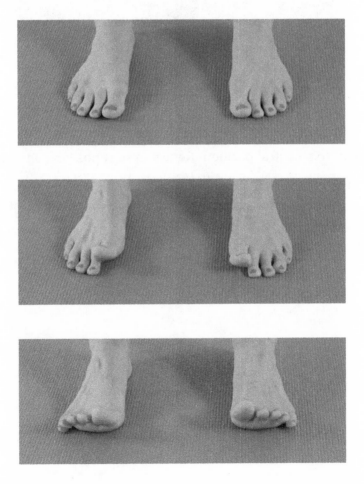

Arch domers/short foot exercise:

Sit in a chair with your feet flat on the ground. Begin with your foot turned out.

Increase the height of your arch by actively attempting to lift your arch, and pull the ball of your foot toward the heel without flexing or moving the toes.

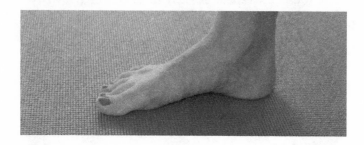

While maintaining the contraction, slide the affected foot across the floor to a neutral position. Return to start position, and repeat. As a progression, perform the previously described arch domer. Upon reaching a neutral position, lift the inside of your foot off of the ground while still maintaining contact of the outside of your foot with the ground.

2. Bridging

One mistake many women make when addressing core and hip strength is to stiffen the spine and over-brace. Bracing is important in certain situations, like when lifting heavy weights and doing power moves. However, for most exercises, the deep core muscle team works best when there is less stiffness and some movement.

Bridging is a great introductory exercise to coordinate pelvic and spinal mobility with core and hip work. It also brings the hips higher than the shoulders, which is helpful during pregnancy, to relieve some of the pressure that the growing fetus places on the spine and pelvic floor.

Lie on your back with your knees bent and your feet flat on the floor. Find your neutral pelvis, or a comfortable position where your back is not excessively arched or tucked. For a full description of neutral pelvis, see Chapter 11.

Take a preparatory breath and activate the pelvic floor muscles on the exhale.

Begin another breath. As you exhale, activate the pelvic floor, feeling the abdominals flatten as they also engage. Begin to tip your pelvis toward your face, allowing the spine to temporarily flatten.

Slowly roll up off of the floor, starting with the hips and pelvis and moving to the spine, one vertebra at a time. Keep equal weight on both legs, and keep the abdominal muscles and pelvic floor working.

Take another breath, and as you exhale, roll down one vertebra at a time.

Repeat 10-15 times.

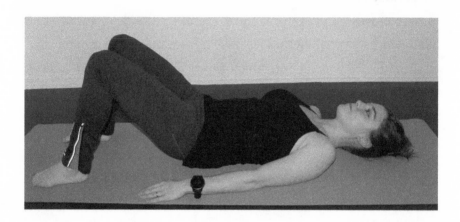

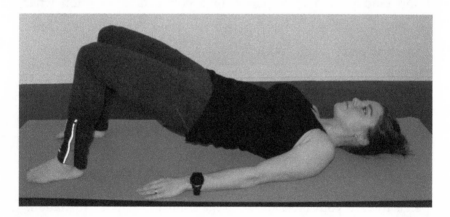

3. Side-Lying Leg Lifts

The side-lying position is a more challenging way to activate the deep core, maintain a neutral pelvis, and introduce movement of the limbs. In the leg lift, the hip muscles—namely the gluteus medius—work to lift the leg. The gluteus medius is responsible for control of the hips and pelvis when in the standing position. Retraining the hip muscles in the side-lying position is a good starting point as you work up to standing exercises for the hips prior to returning to running postnatally.

Lie on one side. Your shoulders and hips should be stacked over each other, and your body should be in a straight line. The best way to do this is to use the long edge of a mat or a wall for reference. You can position yourself parallel to the edge of the mat or parallel to the wall. Bend your bottom knee to improve balance.

Find a neutral pelvis position, which means that the pelvis is not excessively arched or tucked. Your back should not be arched. Your pelvis should not be tucked under with a flat back. You should not feel any pain or discomfort in this position.

Take one breath to prepare. On the next exhale, activate the pelvic floor muscles and lift the top leg about 12 inches. The toes should point toward the front.

Inhale to lower the leg, and repeat on the next exhale. You should feel this on the outside of the hip.

For more of a challenge, prop up onto your forearm. In the propped position, your elbow should line up directly under your shoulder to minimize stress through the arm.

As pregnancy advances, it may be more difficult to prop up due to the weight of your growing abdomen. You may try to use a pillow under the abdomen for support, or you may modify the exercise by lying flat on your side.

Repeat 10-20 times, and then switch sides.

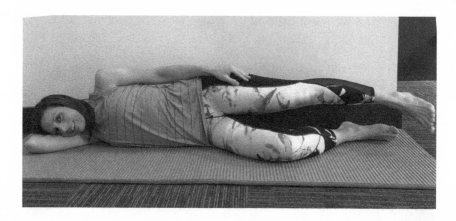

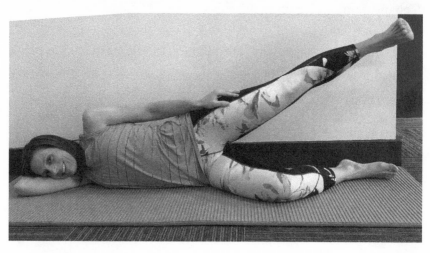

If you are not feeling this exercise on the outside of your hip, it might be too difficult. Try lying with the backside of your body against the wall. Your shoulders, bottom butt cheek, and top leg should all be touching the wall. Bend your bottom leg so that your foot is touching the wall.

Take one breath to prepare. On the next exhale, activate your pelvic floor muscle, and push your top leg into the wall. Then, lift your leg about 12 inches. Your toes should point forward.

Inhale to lower the leg.

Repeat 10-20 times, and then switch sides.

4. Quadruped Hip Extension

As stated, working in the all-fours position is beneficial in pregnancy (see cat/cow exercise). One additional benefit of this position is that it is a good way to address core control and to coordinate arm and leg movements. Lifting a leg to activate the gluteal muscles also challenges core control, as it introduces a degree of instability to the exercise.

Start on your hands and knees. Find a neutral pelvis, lining up your shoulders over your hands and your hips over your knees. For each movement, the trunk should remain in a neutral position, with minimal rotation as the leg moves.

Take a preparatory breath and activate the pelvic floor muscles on the exhale. On the next breath, inhale as you reach one leg behind you, parallel to the floor and no higher than your torso.

Exhale to bend your hip and knee, bringing your leg under you toward your chest.

Repeat with the opposite leg, alternating sides.

Repeat 10 times on each side.

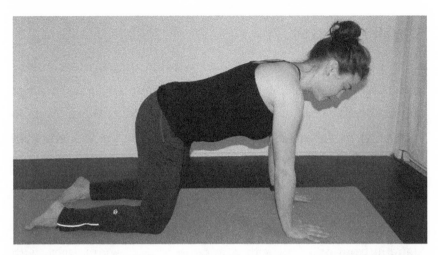

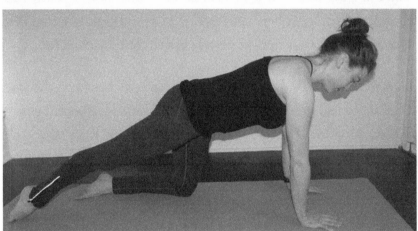

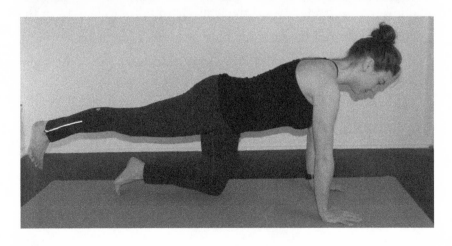

5. Wall Push-Ups

As pregnancy advances, it may become difficult to continue exercising in a plank position. You can continue plank exercises and push-ups on your hands and knees, however. If exercising in a kneeling plank causes knee or wrist pain, or there is any pain or discomfort in the low back or abdomen, a good alternative to address shoulder, chest. and upper extremity strength is a wall push-up.

Stand in front of a wall with your feet shoulder-width apart, with equal weight on your heels and toes. Find neutral pelvis in standing, so that your pelvis is not excessively arched or tucked under.

Lean forward from your ankles, and place your hands on the wall. They should be perpendicular to your body and level with the front of your shoulders. Do not round or arch your back. Keep your chest lifted. You should be able to breathe comfortably in this position.

Take a preparatory breath and activate your pelvic floor muscles on the exhale. On the next breath, inhale as you bend your elbows and lower your body toward the wall. Be mindful to lean from the ankles, and do not flex at your hips or bend your trunk forward. Your shoulder blades should move toward the midline of the back, and toward each other.

As you exhale, press into the wall to separate your shoulder blades, and straighten your elbows in a push-up motion. Maintain a neutral pelvis, and be careful not to round or arch your back. Your elbows should remain close to your trunk through the entire exercise.

Repeat 10-20 times.

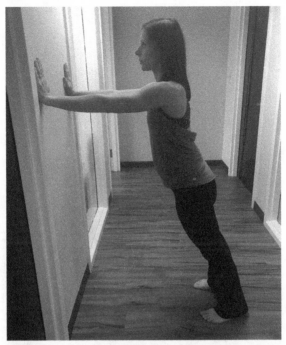

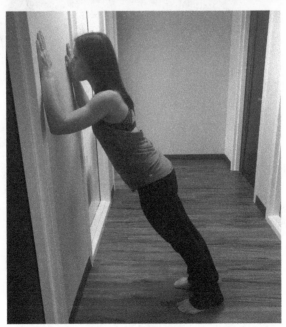

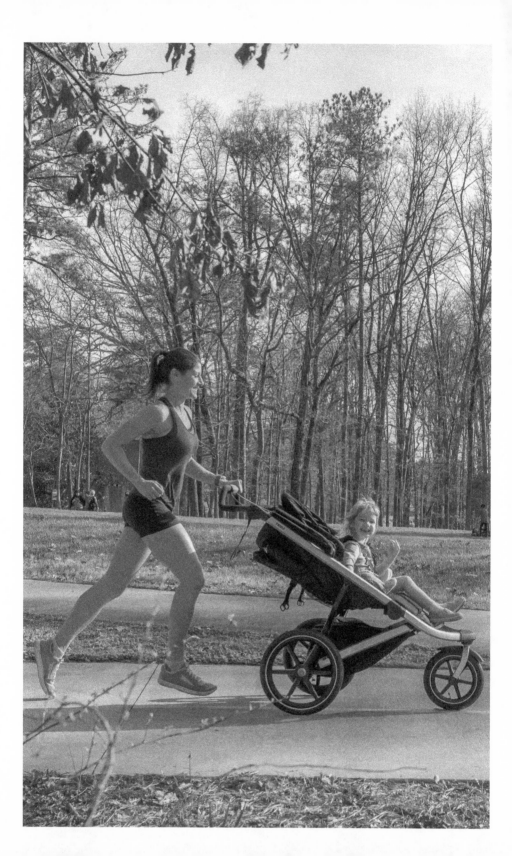

Part Two:
Postpartum

$$\underline{7}$$

Dispelling Postpartum Running Myths

Myth 1:

If you run while breastfeeding, your milk will dry up.

Truth:

Milk production is driven by a feed-forward mechanism involving stimulation of the breasts (by the nursing baby) and hormones. In other words, the more the nipples are stimulated by sucking, the more milk produced. Another driver is caloric intake. Calories must be available to provide energy for milk production. Running burns calories. Remember you will have to replenish your calories in order to maintain milk production. Bottom line: nutrition matters. If milk production is low, hydrate and increase caloric intake as a first intervention.

Myth 2:

After I have a baby, I will have to get used to peeing when I run.

Truth:

Urinary leakage postpartum is common but not normal. Continued leaking that does not change or that increases in frequency or severity is a sign that something is wrong. Seek out a pelvic health PT for help. Don't just tell yourself, "Oh well, this is what happens!" Retraining the pelvic floor muscles while coordinating pelvic floor muscle contractions with breathing and movements—such as jumping—can help eliminate leaking with running.

Myth 3:

Diastasis recti can only be fixed with surgery.

Truth:

As mentioned, diastasis recti is a common occurrence in pregnancy and often will resolve on its own after delivery. It is a problem of fascia stretching and the muscles being unable to control tension as force is applied, such as when lifting weights, doing abdominal exercises, or running and jumping. Many women with diastasis recti improve with appropriate exercises targeting abdominal muscle function and coordination of the deep core muscles. Return to high-impact exercise is possible once these exercises are mastered and the tissue is able to respond to more challenging movements. If you feel like you have a diastasis recti, seek out help from a pelvic health physical therapist who works with postpartum women.

WHAT YOU NEED TO KNOW:

» You had a baby! You are amazing!

» Practice diaphragmatic breathing.

» Once you are postpartum, you are always postpartum.

» During the first six to eight weeks postpartum, there will be a lot of bleeding. If bleeding increases or is excessive, you might be exerting yourself too much.

» Breastfeeding can be painful initially. There are several products that help soothe the pain.

» Place nursing pads in your sports bra in order to decrease the friction on the nipple and to prevent leakage if you produce a large amount of milk.

» You are at a higher risk for stress fractures while you are breastfeeding.

8

The Postpartum Runner

DEFINING POSTPARTUM

Merriam-Webster defines postpartum as, "occurring in or being the period following childbirth." Commonly, this time period is considered to be six weeks, as the postpartum OB/GYN checkup occurs at the six-week mark following childbirth. The Family and Medical Leave Act (FMLA), however, requires eligible employers to provide up to twelve weeks of unpaid leave following childbirth. Therefore, some consider *this* period of time to be postpartum.

Many health care providers also refer to the "fourth trimester" of pregnancy, which would be thirteen weeks following delivery. During this time, mothers have increased physical and emotional needs that should be addressed by a variety of health care providers. In 2018, ACOG created a committee statement, finally recognizing the fourth trimester as an entity, and called upon professionals to rise up and improve the standard of care for postpartum women[34].

In our experience as physical therapists, we believe that once a woman is postpartum, she is always postpartum. Regardless of the length of time used to define the postpartum period, there is one truth worth remembering:

The body undergoes tremendous change and adaptation throughout pregnancy. While it may then change and adapt to no longer being pregnant, it will never be the same as it once was.

That is not to say that women's bodies are not capable; in fact, just the opposite is true. Women are strong; their bodies can meet the demands of raising children, staying active, and training for physical activity, such as running. However, respecting the natural process of healing after childbirth is paramount. Returning to activity postnatally is an example of where slow and steady wins the race, literally and figuratively. If a woman doesn't respect her body during this time, she may be at higher risk for injury later.

INITIAL POSTPARTUM PERIOD

In the first days and weeks following delivery, it is important to let the tissues of the pelvis and vagina rest and heal. During this time, bleeding is normal and common.

However, increased or an excessive volume of blood may be a sign of overexertion. The perineum is often red and/or swollen, and if there was tearing or an episiotomy during childbirth, the incision needs time to heal.

Acceptable movements during the first postpartum month include pelvic tilts, submaximal pelvic floor contractions, and deep breathing. In most cases, short walks (up to fifteen minutes) are beneficial. However, if there are pregnancy/postnatal complications, such as pre-eclampsia, bed rest, or cardiac complications, or if pulmonary embolism occurred, it is important to obtain clearance from the OB/GYN before starting any type of exercise.

By six to eight weeks postpartum, the uterus and vagina have returned to their pre-pregnancy size[27]. It is around this time that women usually return to the OB/GYN for their postpartum check-up. If there are no complications from the delivery, they are typically given a green light to slowly resume their previous level of activity.

RECOVERY FROM C-SECTION

In American culture, women are expected to get up and get moving immediately following childbirth. In the case of a cesarean section, this may not be possible. A cesarean section is major abdominal surgery, after all. To enter the uterus, the surgeon must cut through the abdominal wall first, and then make another incision into the uterus. As with other surgeries, recovery is typically six to eight weeks.

Starting vigorous exercise before the incisions heal may lead to bleeding, dehiscence (the scar coming apart), and pain. Deep breathing and gentle pelvic floor contractions are acceptable in the days following a C-section. Walking upright will help circulation and scar mobility.

Mothers should respect the healing time with regard to exercise, as moms typically are also undergoing other physical stresses associated with the care of a newborn, and possibly older children. Most OB/GYNs will recommend waiting until the postpartum checkup to begin running and other high-intensity exercise. As a reminder, returning to physical activity post-delivery should occur at a slow pace.

Physical status during pregnancy, labor and delivery experience, and life demands in the early postnatal period will all affect the pace and timing of return to activity.

This will be discussed in further detail later.

BREASTFEEDING

Society places a lot of pressure on women to breastfeed their babies. We believe that breastfeeding is optional for all moms. If you decide that breastfeeding is not right for you, do not beat yourself up about it or feel like you are doing something that is not as beneficial for your baby. If you decide that breastfeeding is right for you and your baby, then read on. Breastfeeding can range from uncomfortable to painful at first. If you can make it through the first few days or weeks, it usually gets much easier. Your nipples can become raw and sore, and may even bleed at times, however. This can be very discouraging, but be aware that there are many products available to help decrease the pain of breastfeeding. Some of these products include lanolin gel, to put on the nipples, and nipple guards.

Lactation is the process by which women produce milk for their babies. It is driven by hormonal changes, starting with the delivery of the baby and placenta. Milk production in the breasts is a feed-forward mechanism: sucking on the nipple (or a sucking sensation, such as with a breast pump) is a stimulus that drives the continued production of milk in the breasts.

The hormones that control milk production are prolactin and oxytocin. Women who are lactating have decreased levels of estrogen and progesterone. While a mom is breastfeeding, her breasts can weigh three pounds more than when she is not pregnant or nursing. Three additional pounds each! Breast weight, hormone levels, and mom's posture during feeding can all affect how a woman's body responds to nursing. The additional weight of the breasts and rounding of the thorax can also affect her posture and comfort while running.

In addition, increased breast size may affect the ability of the ribs to expand with breathing, reducing oxygen efficiency with exercise. Joint laxity typically does not resolve until breastfeeding has ceased[27]. A supportive sports bra and nursing pads can be your best friends at this point. The more supported the breasts are, the less painful running will be. Additionally, placing nursing pads inside of your sports bra will help decrease the friction on the nipple and make it less painful. The nursing pads can also be useful if you produce excessive amounts of milk, as they can help decrease the chances of getting milk spots on the front of your shirt.

Bone mineral density (BMD) is also affected in the postpartum period, particularly with breastfeeding. This occurs because the calcium in the mother's bones is mobilized to meet the increased demand for calcium in the mother's milk[41].

Hormonal changes, such as high prolactin and low estrogen levels, promote bone resorption[41]. Estrogen levels remain low until the return of menses. Unfortunately, taking calcium supplements has not been found to increase BMD during breastfeeding[41-44].

During breastfeeding, bone loss is one to three percent per month. The pelvis, hip joint, and lumbar spine are composed of trabecular bone, which is less-dense bone material, and the site of bone development and reabsorption. Three to nine percent of maternal bone loss occurs at trabecular-rich sites, such as the hip and lumbar spine[41-43]. In most women, BMD loss is reversed with cessation of breastfeeding and may return to baseline in twelve to eighteen months. However, in some cases, complete recovery may not occur[42]. BMD loss is associated with osteopenia and osteoporosis later in life, and is a factor in bone stress injuries, such as stress reactions and stress fractures among runners[42,45,46]. All of this is to say that there is a high risk for stress fractures postpartum, and especially when you are breastfeeding.

ENERGY & REST

The energy needs of a breastfeeding mom are greater than those of a pregnant woman[47,48]. Sleep and nutrition are of utmost importance during this time. Fatigue is one of the one most common complaints among postpartum mothers[49]. Women may need an additional 500 calories per day for adequate milk production and energy needs.

With intense activity, such as running, she may require an even greater caloric intake[48]. Hydration may be an issue as well, with the necessary increased fluid requirements. It is a myth that exercise inhibits milk production; if the mother is getting adequate food and fluid to account for the extra water and calorie loss with running or exercise, she will be able to maintain her milk supply. In fact, if milk supply decreases with increased activity, that may be a sign that it is necessary to increase calories and/or fluids consumed.

As mentioned previously, adequate rest is a priority during the early postpartum weeks. Sleep is a time of recovery for the body, and especially the muscular system, as muscle recovery occurs during times of relative rest. If a mother is taking care of her family and home, as well as nursing and exercising, that leaves little time for rest.

Depending on her work status, she may take on job demands as well, even in the first three months following delivery. Lack of sleep may trigger the production of cortisol, a hormone involved in the stress response. Elevated cortisol may be a temporary benefit, as it is responsible for the "fight or flight" response that accompanies increased stress. However, chronically elevated stress levels and cortisol can have a detrimental effect on how the body responds to exercise. Instead of feeling energized, fit, and strong, a mom may instead feel lethargic, sore, and exhausted. Optimal muscle recovery may be inhibited, and over time, this could lead to injury, such as unresolved musculoskeletal pain. Signs of overtraining may appear sooner, as the nervous system tries to send the body a signal to slow down.

Clinical signs and symptoms of overtraining to be aware of include: decreased training pleasure, sleep disturbances, fatigue, vulnerability to respiratory infections, memory disturbances, decrease in professional efficacy, irritability, digestive disturbances, muscle soreness, and loss of training desire[50]. As a new mom, you may experience many of these symptoms, whether you are training or not. Be aware, and if you are experiencing one or more as you increase your exercise, it should be a red flag that you are doing too much.

The best way to control the cortisol response is to get adequate rest. This may mean taking a nap with the baby in the afternoon, enlisting your partner to help with nighttime feedings, finding stretches of time to dedicate to self-care—including rest—and engaging in mindfulness and other low-energy, pleasurable activities. This may also mean delaying your return to longer runs until the baby is able to sleep for longer stretches during the night.

Another struggle that can get in the way of running is simply getting used to the "new normal." Both new moms and moms with other children in the home have to make some adjustments. The presence of a new baby can disrupt the daily flow, and it may take some time until balance is restored. New challenges, such as coordinating carpools, helping with homework, getting to and from school or work, and attending to housekeeping needs while caring for a newborn may all get in the way of finding time to exercise. It is common for moms to give up sleep to allow themselves to get everything accomplished and still be able to work out. This creates stress in addition to fatigue, however, and as already mentioned, both can be detrimental to her attempts to return to exercise. It is important to remember that new routines take time to establish.

Incorporating short periods of specific physical activity throughout the day or week can help establish an exercise routine while the family is working together to come up with the best system for everyone. These routines may include drills, strength work, flexibility, and even brief runs. Appropriate drills and return to running programs will be discussed later.

Some women have a more difficult time adjusting to changing schedules, lifestyles, and care demands. Without a doubt, it can be overwhelming. Asking for help is normal, and we encourage this. Local moms' groups, friends, and family may also be able to provide support and guidance. If this is not enough, professionals such as psychologists and life coaches can provide tools and support to create more balance.

Exercise is a form of stress relief; creating more stress and fatigue in order to keep exercising is counterproductive.

EXERCISE RECOMMENDATIONS

The American College of Sports Medicine recommends 150 minutes of exercise weekly, at a moderate pace, for cardiovascular health. While this may not seem like a lot to runners accustomed to long distances, it is a good starting point when returning to regular exercise. The other good news is that the 150 minutes do not need to occur in long stretches or blocks of time.

Initially, it may be easier to run or jog for 30 minutes twice a day instead of one hour once a day. It also could make sense to run for 60 minutes three times a week instead of every day. Small bouts of exercise mixed with sufficient sleep will improve recovery and minimize the risk for injury and overtraining at first, until the time when the baby is old enough to be in a jogging stroller or sleeping longer at night. See Chapters 12 and 13 for ways to modify your exercise program, as well as return-to-running programs for runners that ran a little throughout pregnancy, consistently through pregnancy, or who are new to running altogether.

WHAT YOU NEED TO KNOW:

» Peeing yourself is common but not normal; if you are leaking even a little bit, seek out help.

» There are people and resources to help you recover from pelvic floor dysfunction.

» Pelvic floor dysfunction can occur even if you have a C-section.

» Pelvic floor dysfunction can occur several years after having a baby.

» Taking the time in the early postpartum period to address your pelvic floor health can prevent problems later in life.

» Physical therapy and exercise are effective ways to manage impairments from pelvic floor dysfunction and diastasis recti abdominis.

9

Common Pelvic Floor Dysfunctions

The delivery of a baby is not only a special time emotionally, but it is also a tremendous physical effort. The female body is built to withstand the trauma of delivery. Unfortunately, the process of labor and delivery is not without risk, for both vaginal deliveries and cesarean sections. As mentioned, the bony pelvis, pelvic floor muscles, and associated soft tissue undergo a tremendous amount of stretch and change throughout pregnancy. This is in an effort to prepare the body for labor and delivery. During labor and delivery, the pelvic floor muscles can stretch to two to three times their resting length[51]. Despite these adaptations, this region of the body is at an increased risk for injury and dysfunction long after pregnancy and delivery.

Some of the risks for pelvic floor dysfunction following a vaginal delivery include:

- Instrument-assisted delivery—forceps or vacuum
- Perineal tearing
- Episiotomy
- Prolonged second stage of labor—the "push" phase of labor that can extend for several hours

Electing to have a C-section or undergoing an emergency C-section does not make you exempt from postpartum pelvic floor dysfunction. Changing biomechanics, muscle length and function, increased weight of a growing baby and uterus, and a history of previous pregnancies and/or vaginal deliveries may also contribute to pelvic floor dysfunction following a cesarean delivery. If you experienced pushing prior to receiving a C-section, the time spent in the second stage of labor may also present a risk for future injury.

Additionally, it is important to remember that this is major surgery. Initial healing of scar tissue may be difficult and painful. The scarring is not just in the abdomen, either; the doctor must also cut into the uterus to deliver the baby. This is often forgotten as women are sent home after delivery with little instruction on how to recover from surgery, while simultaneously caring for a newborn. Taking time to care for yourself is paramount, and doing so will minimize your risk for long-term pelvic floor dysfunction, as well as other musculoskeletal disorders. Ignoring the process of healing from surgery can lead to difficulty with scar healing, pain, and ultimately, will result in a longer wait to return to daily activity and exercise.

Impaired pelvic floor function is associated with postpartum musculoskeletal problems, such as low back pain[52-55]. It is well known that women experience low back pain (LBP) and pelvic girdle pain (PGP) during and following pregnancy. To be exact, 50 percent of women experience LBP or PGP during pregnancy, and many of them continue to experience pain in the postnatal period[56].

One study showed a stronger association between low back pain and incontinence than between low back pain and obesity or physical activity[54]. This is significant because it highlights the relationship between the muscles of the low back, abdomen, and pelvic floor. We discuss postpartum low back pain in more detail in Chapter 10, but we want to highlight here how the pelvic floor muscles are involved in low back pain, and emphasize that they should not be ignored during the recovery process.

What is not discussed as widely as low back pain is the incidence of pelvic floor dysfunction, which includes problems such as urinary and fecal incontinence, pelvic organ prolapse, and pelvic pain. In fact, many women do not experience these problems until years following childbirth. They begin to regard things such as incontinence and urinary leakage as a "normal" part of aging, or a normal consequence of giving birth. According to Dietz and Lanzarone, up to 36 percent of vaginal deliveries are associated with a partial or complete tear of the levator ani muscle group[38]. The levator ani is a group of muscles whose primary functions include support of the pelvic organs and trunk stability. Like other muscles in the body, the pelvic floor muscles need time to heal, or their function can be compromised in the long term.

The most common postpartum disorders of the pelvic floor are known as supportive pelvic floor disorders. This means that the pelvic floor muscles are unable to provide adequate support and control for the pelvic organs, or that they struggle to regulate urination and defecation. There are many factors that may lead to supportive pelvic floor dysfunction. The easiest way to think about the pelvic floor is if it were a pressure system. Recall that the pelvic floor muscles interact as a team with the abdominals, low back, and diaphragm to help control intra-abdominal pressure (IAP). Injury to the pelvic floor, such as tearing or stretching during delivery, may reduce the ability of the pelvic floor muscles to generate sufficient force to counteract changes in IAP. Likewise, postural changes, new movement strategies, and even muscle fatigue can affect the ability of the pelvic floor muscles to control IAP. Examples of supportive pelvic floor dysfunction are stress urinary incontinence (SUI) and pelvic organ prolapse (POP).

STRESS URINARY INCONTINENCE (SUI)

A common misconception of incontinence is that it involves a complete loss of control of the bladder and urethra and results in significant urine loss. SUI is defined by the International Continence Society as a "complaint of involuntary loss of urine on effort or physical exertion, including sporting activities etc., or on sneezing or coughing[57]." Many people believe that occasional leakage, or leaking only with coughing, sneezing, running, jumping, etc. is normal in women who have given birth.

Unfortunately, American society and culture has completely normalized this disorder. While SUI is common, affecting up to one third of women with children, it is not a normal postpartum occurrence[58].

Urinary continence is controlled by the bladder and the PFM—namely the muscles and connective tissue surrounding the urethra[59]. The bladder is a smooth muscle; when it fills, the muscle stretches until it signals that it is time to empty. The brain tells the bladder muscle to contract and the PFM to relax to allow urine to pass. If the nervous system determines it is not time to urinate, the PFM contracts and the bladder remains relaxed. In order for this to occur, there must be a coordinated effort of the muscles of the abdomen, low back, diaphragm, and PFM, in addition to tension in the pelvic fascia and coordinated timing.

In other words, this all has to occur at just the right time, with just the right amount of force to control urethral pressure. The more pressure that is exerted onto the urethra and pelvic floor muscles by the abdomen and bladder, such as with coughing, sneezing, or weight-bearing/impact (jumping or running), the more force required by the PFM to counteract this pressure and prevent leakage. Sustained loading on the PFM, such as during pregnancy, and more forceful stretch of the PFM, such as during childbirth, can alter the ability of the PFM to counteract high loads, quick loading, or sustained load over time, leading to SUI.

While the thought of having to live a life with SUI may present a picture of doom and gloom, the good news is that the PFM can be retrained and the continence mechanism restored. Multiple studies show the efficacy of PFM retraining to prevent long-term SUI following childbirth. Retraining the PFM starts with building awareness of the muscles and the ability to contract them and close the urethra.

These are known as Kegel exercises, named for the man who first started using them with patients.

Once a woman is successfully able to contract and fully relax the PFM, training advances to working on fast-versus-slow contractions, sustained holds, and quick, repeated contractions. She can then learn how to incorporate the PFM into functional activities, such as walking, squatting, climbing stairs, bending, and lifting. The final step of retraining the PFM involves teaching the muscles how to respond to the loading and impact that occurs with sport activity, such as running. The PFM are made up of both fast- and slow-twitch fibers, and therefore, both the strength and endurance components of these muscles should be trained.

Additionally, the PFM should be trained in coordination with the diaphragm, low back, and abdominal muscles. Rarely in our bodies do muscles work in isolation, and the pelvic floor is no exception. Learning how to contract and relax the PFM is the first step, followed by coordinating the glutes, abs, and even breathing. A long-term goal to improve PFM function and minimize incontinence symptoms involves creating an exercise program that incorporates multiple muscle groups and body movements, and pays special attention to how the PFM are responding to high impact loading.

Leaking of urine during or after exercise or any activity is a sign that load is too great or mechanics are not right. Exercises can take some modifying and fine tuning. We will discuss more specific exercises in Chapter 12.

PELVIC ORGAN PROLAPSE (POP)

By definition, POP is the descent of the anterior or posterior vaginal wall, the apex of the vagina, or the uterus. It is very common after childbirth and in older women. The incidence of POP is about 40 percent[60]. Other names for POP include cystocele, urethrocele, enterocele, and rectocele. Regardless of the terminology, the mechanism is the same: There is not enough integrity of the soft-tissue structures in the pelvis to support the pelvic organs.

As is the case with SUI, POP can occur as a result of insufficient muscle strength/function, or it may be due to the inability of the pelvic soft tissue to withstand increasing intra-abdominal pressure. The result is an outpouching of the vaginal tissue into the vaginal canal, and possibly past the hymen, where it may become visible. Symptoms of POP include feelings of pelvic pressure, and like something is "falling out of the vagina." Pain, discomfort, impaired bowel and bladder function, and impaired sexual function may also coexist with POP. Many women undergo surgery to correct POP because they are told it is the only way to resolve symptoms. Unfortunately, up to a third of surgeries to correct POP fail.

Luckily, there are other ways to manage POP and mitigate symptoms without surgical intervention.

One non-surgical intervention for POP is a device called a pessary. A pessary is an insertable device that fits into the vagina. Its purpose is to counteract the increased pressure leading to prolapse and prevent descent of the pelvic organs. Pessaries can be helpful, though they are not "one size fits all," and it can be difficult to find a good fit. Sometimes, women can wear a pessary during high-impact/high-pressure activities, such as running, jumping, lifting weights, carrying children, and housework, and then remove it for less strenuous activities. Other pessaries stay in place for longer periods of time. A pessary is a good temporary solution to manage mild to moderate POP. If you think you would benefit from a pessary, you can discuss it with your physical therapist, who may be able to make a recommendation. However, in the United States, only doctors can prescribe or fit patients for pessaries.

Another way to manage and even reduce symptoms of POP in mild to moderate cases is through exercise. Exercises for POP include PFM retraining and management of intra-abdominal pressure. Similar to SUI, instruction in specific exercises to address the strength and function of the pelvic floor and the supporting musculature (diaphragm, low back, and abdominals) is beneficial for improving POP symptoms. Addressing posture, alignment, strength, motor control, and coordination is an integral part of an exercise program to improve symptoms of POP. Several studies support PFM retraining as a way to reduce the severity of POP symptoms[60,61]. More information on exercises to improve POP symptoms will be provided in Chapter 12.

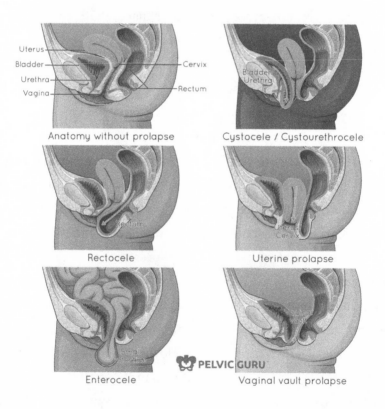

Pelvic Organ Prolapse, courtesy of Pelvic Guru

PELVIC PAIN

Women experience pelvic pain following childbirth for a variety of reasons. The process of labor and delivery can be painful due to the widening of the pelvis and the stretching of related soft-tissue structures. Yet pain is a normal part of the healing process. Pain that lasts longer than two months, however, is not a normal occurrence, and should be addressed by a doctor. If at any time in the early postnatal period you experience pain with fever, redness, warmth, or excessive bleeding, it is imperative that you see a doctor immediately. These could be signs of a hemorrhage or an infection.

After several weeks, the tissue in the perineum should be healed. The doctor or midwife typically assesses this at the six-week postnatal visit. Factors that may impact soft-tissue healing include tears, episiotomy scars, and delayed C-section scar healing. Lack of sleep, dehydration, and inadequate nutrition may also delay tissue healing.

The musculoskeletal system can also be a source of postpartum pelvic pain. Trauma to the joints and muscles in the pelvis can linger for weeks and even months following delivery. Pain in the sacroiliac joints and pubic symphysis is known as pelvic girdle pain (PGP). Persistent musculoskeletal pain, including PGP, is not normal and should be addressed by a physician or a physical therapist.

Pubic symphysis dysfunction occurs as a result of separation of the joint. A severe separation of more than nine millimeters is considered a dislocation. While rare, it can occur postpartum. Women who experience this type of dysfunction are typically not able to bear weight and have great difficulty walking and moving in bed. Physical therapy is indicated to help women learn how to move and walk, and to train women in the use of a walker as the joint is healing. Braces and belts are helpful supports to the pubic symphysis during the acute recovery phase to minimize excessive movement at the joint and reduce pain with walking and position changes, such as getting in and out of bed or a chair.

Another common type of PGP is sacroiliac joint (SIJ) pain. This can also impact overall mobility and function. The cause of SIJ pain in the postnatal period is unknown, but some studies suggest that the trauma of labor and delivery is one potential contributor to SIJ pain. The presence of SIJ pain is thought to relate to difficulty with transferring load through the pelvis[62]. This may lead to difficulty not only with walking and childcare activities, but also with return to exercise.

Tailbone pain, also known as coccydynia, may occur following a vaginal delivery. It is typically caused by birthing position and pressure on the tailbone while pushing during labor. Coccydynia contributes to pain with sitting, and even standing and walking. It may cause painful bowel movements as well.

Physical therapy interventions, including manual therapy and muscle retraining, are effective ways to treat postnatal PGP and musculoskeletal pain in other areas of the body[62]. In addition to exercise instruction and hands-on techniques, physical therapists provide education about what to expect during recovery and how to modify activities to minimize pain and discomfort throughout each phase of rehabilitation. Regardless of the type of exercises prescribed, education is a necessary part of rehabilitation for postnatal pelvic and pelvic girdle pain.

DIASTASIS RECTI ABDOMINIS (DRA)

DRA is not technically a type of pelvic floor dysfunction, but rather an abdominal impairment. It is the separation of the linea alba that occurs in pregnancy. The linea alba is the connective tissue that sits between the two rectus abdominis muscles in the midline of the abdomen. During pregnancy, the abdominal muscles stretch and expand as the uterus grows. It is common for the connective tissue to stretch and sometimes tear. In fact, two-thirds of pregnant women are affected by DRA by the third trimester. Although 60 percent of women with DRA will recover by six months postpartum, those who do not may deal with problems, including impaired abdominal and core strength, low back pain, urinary incontinence, and pelvic organ prolapse[30].

One study found that two-thirds of women seeking help for postnatal SUI and POP also had DRA present on examination, even if they were not aware of it[63]. This is not enough to definitively say that one causes the other; however, both PFD and DRA are often seen together. Considering the anatomy and relationship of the pelvic floor and abdominal muscles (remember, they make up part of the deep core), it makes sense that PFD and DRA would occur simultaneously.

Historically, treating DRA has focused on "closing the gap," or using exercise and abdominal binders to help the tear repair itself. Women have been told to avoid crunches, sit-ups, planks, and other exercises that involve isolated contractions of the rectus abdominus in favor of "abdominal bracing" strategies more focused on activating the transversus abdominus. Many doctors advocate for surgery, claiming this is the only way to fix the DRA. The result is a great deal of misinformation about DRA, the prognosis, and what women can and cannot do from an exercise and activity standpoint. More recent studies show that perhaps "closing the gap" should not be the goal of rehabilitation, but instead, the objective should be to restore the ability to create tension across the abdominal fascia (Lee, 2016). This school of thought contends that there is a difference between appearance and function; while the width of the split may not disappear completely, the tear itself can be controlled from a depth perspective by retraining the core. This means that a woman with DRA can be taught how to coordinate the effort of the deep core muscles, including the diaphragm, abdominals, and PFM, and then work to gradually increase load and movement to retrain the capacity of the muscles to support the demands of exercise and life.

There is not a clear answer as to which exercises are best to treat DRA, or if a woman will end up needing surgery. The best approach to treatment of DRA, similar to POP, is one that manages the pressure in the abdomen and minimizes the tissues bulging out (also known as "doming") when effort is exerted. This involves understanding how to retrain the muscles and slowly adding movements, different positions, and varying degrees of stress to the tissues without creating more pressure.

Doming, or bulging of the abdominal contents upon exertion, is a sign that the effort or load is too great and should be avoided when possible. Women who have severe DRA may benefit from abdominal braces or binders to provide external support as the muscles are healing. The use of a binder as a long-term strategy is not advised, however, as it may discourage the muscles from working to their maximal capacity. Physical therapists who work with postnatal women are well equipped to assess DRA and determine the best treatment strategy for each individual.

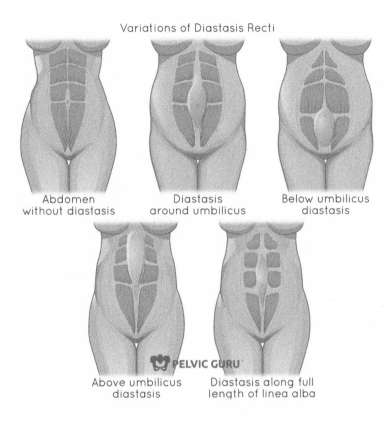

Diastasis Recti Abdominis, courtesy of Pelvic Guru

WHAT YOU NEED TO KNOW:

» Injuries to the postpartum runner can occur during pregnancy, during childbirth, or postpartum.

» Many of the injuries postpartum women experience are common amongst all runners; however, the postpartum runner may be at a higher risk.

» Stress fractures are common among women who are breastfeeding.

» Listen to your body, and take it slowly when returning to running.

10

Musculoskeletal Injuries in Postpartum Runners

A runner's foot strikes the ground between 800 and 1,500 times per mile, with forces that are 1.5 to five times his or her body weight. The slower a person runs, the more impact the body will endure over time (i.e.: an eight-minute mile equals approximately 1,400 steps per minute, and a twelve-minute mile equals approximately 1,951 steps per minute). It is no wonder between 19 and 92 percent of runners become injured[4,6,64].

There are some common movement patterns in injured runners observed in research and by clinicians. These patterns occur distally at the foot, and include increased stride length, excessive ankle dorsiflexion or inversion at foot strike, excessive foot eversion, and toe-in and toe-out gait. They also occur more proximally at the hip and knee, such as increased genu varum (knees out) and valgum (knees collapsing in), anterior pelvic tilt, and contralateral pelvic drop.

One of the most common abnormal movement patterns is the combination of excessive hip adduction (hip coming in), internal rotation, and pelvic drop[5]. These patterns can be seen in both men and women. However, postpartum women may be more prone to some of these patterns, having gone through so many physical changes during pregnancy.

Injuries to the postpartum runner can occur as a result of the biomechanical or physiological changes of pregnancy, from labor and delivery or from the psychosocial aspects of caring for children. Running injuries do not only occur in the first or second year postpartum; they may occur years later, secondary to the remaining postural changes and strategies described in Chapter 11. Below, we describe some common injuries that occur, what they feel like, and why they occur. In Chapter 12, we will outline some of the exercises that can help prevent and rehabilitate the injuries described.

PUBIC SYMPHYSIS PAIN

The pubic symphysis is a cartilaginous joint between the two pubic bones that connects the pelvic ring, and it is subject to much stress during pregnancy and childbirth. As discussed in Chapter 9, pubic symphysis pain may occur as a result. Pain in the pubic symphysis may be localized, or it may radiate to the inner thighs, groin, or even low back. Onset of pain is often gradual, but can be sudden in some cases[65]. Pubic symphysis pain can result from ligament laxity, labor, or delivery. Mild pubic symphysis pain may resolve with ice and rest.

More severe pubic symphysis pain may be a result of osteitis pubis. Osteitis pubis is characterized by bony resorption about the symphysis followed by spontaneous re-ossification of the pubic tubercles[65,66]. The pain in the pubic symphysis may initially be mild, but will rapidly progress to severe. Physical therapy can help with osteitis pubis. Treatment should not be limited to the pubic bone itself, but should also include the structures above and below that influence it, such as the lumbar spine, sacroiliac joints, and hips. Treatment of osteitis pubis often focuses on pain relief initially, and then progresses to include balancing joint mobility, muscle strength and endurance, and motor control.

STRESS FRACTURES

Stress fractures in runners most commonly occur in the femur, tibia, and fifth metatarsal (the outside bone of the foot); however, they can also occur in the spine, fibula, pelvis, and sacrum. Stress fractures typically present with sharp pain during weight-bearing activity, such as walking, running, and jumping. They will feel better with rest. Often, muscular tightness in the region of the stress fracture and some associated aching occurs. Stress fractures are a result of weakness in the bone. Stress fractures are multifactorial for runners, particularly postpartum.

Bone mineral density (BMD) is affected in the postpartum period, particularly with breastfeeding. BMD directly relates to calcium in the bones. When a woman is breastfeeding, the calcium in her bones is mobilized to meet the increased demand for calcium in breast milk[41,43]. Additionally, hormonal changes, such as high prolactin and low estrogen levels, promote bone resorption[42]. Estrogen levels remain low until the return of menses, which typically does not occur until a woman stops breastfeeding. Unfortunately, calcium supplements have not been found to increase BMD during breastfeeding[41-43,67].

Maternal bone loss is estimated to be one to three percent per month. In the bones of the hip joint and lumbar spine, the bone loss may be up to nine percent[41,43,44]. In most women, BMD loss is reversed with cessation of breastfeeding, and may return to baseline in twelve to eighteen months. In some cases, however, complete recovery may not occur[42]. BMD loss is associated with osteopenia and osteoporosis later in life, and is a factor in bone stress injuries, such as stress reactions and stress fractures among runners[42,45,46].

Once a stress fracture has occurred, the average healing time is six to eight weeks under good circumstances. This means getting adequate sleep and following a healthy diet with proper nutrition. Most parents of newborns and infants are lucky to get four to six consecutive hours of sleep, however, and are eating takeout or whatever people bring them once the new baby comes home. So, it is realistic to say sleep and nutrition are among the many compromises often made with a new baby. Yet, to heal properly, stress fractures require rest, balanced nutritional intake, possible nutritional counseling, and a review of training habits.

In addition to these basic requirements, many women may also require a period of non-weight bearing, which may include use of a walking boot, a spring plate in the shoe, or crutches, depending on the severity and location of the stress fracture. Physical therapy, functional movement screening, strength training, and gait analysis will also be beneficial when recovering from a stress fracture. Even if you are in a boot, on crutches, or using a spring plate, you can still work on core stability, breathing, posture, and much more while the bone is healing. Taking this route rather than waiting will ultimately get you back to running and life much faster. After all, it's no fun lugging a car seat around while in a boot.

LABRAL TEARS

The labrum is a ring of fibrocartilage that extends from the hip joint, known as the acetabulum (hip socket). The job of the labrum is to deepen the hip socket, help regulate the synovial fluid (lubricant in the joint), protect the articular cartilage, and create more stability and load bearing at the hip[68].

Injury to the labrum can change the mechanics, stability, and health of the hip joint. A labral injury can occur in anyone, especially if the person has a bony abnormality, such as a cam lesion on the femoral head or a pincer lesion on the rim of the acetabulum. Cam or pincer lesions can lead to a condition known as femoroacetabuar impingement (FAI), which can cause hip and groin pain with running. A history of FAI may contribute to the development of a labral tear in the hip joint.

A labral injury will often present with pain in the anterior groin or in a "c-shape," from the anterolateral part of the hip to the posterior lateral portion of the hip. It is often described as "pinching, catching, locking or clicking," and may be accompanied by hip flexor weakness and increased tightness in the anterolateral hip musculature. The pain is typically aggravated by weight bearing, twisting, pivoting, prolonged sitting (especially in a deep chair), walking, running, and using stairs. Hip range of motion will be less in flexion, adduction, and internal rotation[68].

Theories as to why pregnant women end up with labral tears include increased ligament laxity and increased axial load secondary to weight gain and trauma in labor and delivery. During labor and delivery, extreme flexion and internal rotation of the hip that causes

123

pinching of the labrum may occur. The more forceful the position, the more likely there is pinching on the labrum[68]. Many women sustain labral tears as nurses and assistants in the delivery room forcefully place their hips at these end-ranges of motion while they are pushing. In some cases, this position is necessary to ensure the baby's safety during delivery. However, it may be wise to consider other birthing positions (squatting, lying on your side, water birth) to minimize the risk of hip injury during labor and delivery, if it is safe for both you and your baby. Clinicians can test for a labral tear in the patient exam, but to know for sure, it is officially diagnosed with a test called MRA with contrast. The hip joint is injected with dye, and the patient undergoes an MRI. The dye helps the radiologist visualize the hip joint and see whether there is a tear in the labrum.

Physical therapy is an effective way to treat FAI and labral tears. Treatment focuses on restoring normal joint mechanics and balance of the muscles around the hip joint, including the glutes, adductors, and deep hip rotators. In addition, focusing on core control and abdominal and pelvic floor function is paramount to recovery. In certain cases, surgery may be indicated to fully recover from a labral tear.

LOW BACK PAIN

Low back pain is a common dysfunction in men and women in the United States and the most common musculoskeletal injury during pregnancy and postpartum. Many of the biomechanical and physiological changes that occur during pregnancy and remain postpartum can contribute to low back pain. We have already discussed many of these changes. Some of the changes seen in women postpartum include altered muscle activity in the back, hip, and abdominal musculature, ligament laxity, and changes in spinal and pelvic positioning[69].

Low back pain can present in many ways, including aching, burning, pinching, tightness, or sharp pain. It is often located in the back, but might refer into the buttocks or to one or both legs. Sometimes, referral may initially feel like tightness and pulling in one or more of the hamstring muscles, or like burning or pain. Over time, if left untreated, low back pain can make simple, everyday tasks, like picking up children, bending, sleeping, sitting, walking, or running extremely difficult.

The experience of low back pain can be scary, especially if you start to read articles online that discuss severe injuries, such as herniated discs and fractures. The majority of the time, however, low back pain is muscular in nature, or due to altered body mechanics. If you are experiencing low back pain, we suggest seeing a physical therapist for an evaluation. The physical therapist can screen you for any severe situations that would require medical intervention and prescribe specific exercises to address muscle imbalances and mobility impairments. Manual therapy is also effective in many instances, even during pregnancy. Treatment of low back pain in the postpartum runner should include a combination of mobility exercises, breathing and pelvic floor exercises, deep core stability exercises, postural re-education, strengthening, and neuro-muscular control of the trunk and lower extremities. In Chapter 12, we outline many basic exercises that can help prevent or rehabilitate low back pain in postpartum runners.

KNEE PAIN

Knee injuries are the number-one cited injury in runners. They are often the result of weakness in the pelvic girdle or foot structure, poor training habits (overtraining), and knee stiffness, among other things[5,12]. Women who are postpartum may experience knee pain as they attempt to resume running. The musculoskeletal changes of pregnancy and altered gait patterns we have previously discussed make postpartum women susceptible to knee pain.

This is a strong argument for working on the exercises in Chapter 12 before resuming running. Setting up the foundation for good muscle function and counteracting some of the changes that have occurred in pregnancy will help prevent the onset of knee pain as you return to running. The two most common knee injuries in runners are iliotibial band syndrome (ITBS) and patellofemoral pain (PFP). The most abnormal movement patterns associated with knee pain in runners are hip drop, hip adduction, and femoral internal rotation[5], all of which are common postpartum.

ITBS can present with pain that occurs in the hip, lateral thigh, or knee. It can come on slowly over the course of several weeks, or following a single training run. Symptoms are often described as stiffness or swelling at the lateral knee or hip, achiness, sharp pain, inability to straighten the leg fully, pain with descending stairs, pain when the foot hits the ground—either when walking or running—and limping.

PFP can present as aching, clicking, grinding, swelling, or pain in the front of the knee. The aching will often occur following prolonged sitting, with bending or squatting, or when ascending or descending stairs.

A majority of knee injuries can be treated with physical therapy focused on gait mechanics/retraining, strength and neuromuscular control of the hip and pelvic girdle, and proprioception and control of the foot and ankle. Manual therapy to address soft tissue and joint mobility impairments should also be included.

Some simple gait changes that might be helpful include shortening step length during a run or running on stable but softer surfaces, such as a track, treadmill, or grass, to reduce knee stiffness[12]. Increasing cadence by five to 10 percent is another effective intervention to improve knee pain with running.

POSTERIOR THIGH PAIN

Posterior thigh pain (pain in the back of the leg) is another common running injury. It can be caused by several different structures, including the muscles or the lumbar spine. It is frequently a combination of structures that causes the pain. Changes to posture and mechanics during pregnancy make the postpartum runner susceptible to posterior thigh pain as she resumes training. As with lower back pain, in most cases, this is not a medical emergency and can be treated with small changes in gait, specific exercises, and hands-on manual therapy.

A common contributor to posterior thigh pain is the hamstring muscle group. The hamstrings have a direct attachment to not only the bony pelvis, but also to some of the ligaments in the area. Ligament laxity predisposes the hamstrings to additional stress, as these muscles work to maintain pelvic stability in addition to their role in facilitating hip and knee movement. Hamstring injuries will typically be more painful when running uphill, faster running, bending forward, straightening or bending the knee, and walking.

If you feel you are experiencing hamstring pain, do not overstretch the muscle. This could make it worse. One of the most important things that can be done for chronic hamstring issues is eccentric exercise. Eccentric exercises allow the muscles to work as they are lengthening and accepting load, which is different than a concentric, or shortening, contraction. Examples of eccentric exercises in Chapter 12 include ball hamstring curls and one-leg dead lifts. Adding eccentric exercises to your regular strength routine will better prepare your hamstrings for running.

One muscle that can mimic hamstring pain is the obturator internus muscle. The obturator internus is a hip rotator and pelvic floor muscle. A small part of the muscle can be located on the lateral hip, but the majority of its surface area is internal. Changes in pelvic mobility and alignment, altered gait mechanics, and the experience of labor and delivery can predispose women to obturator internus dysfunction.

Because of its location on the inside of the pelvis, it is often missed in a basic evaluation of the hip joint or lumbar spine and pelvis. A pelvic health physical therapist is able to adequately assess this muscle. The easiest way to treat this muscle is to perform a manual release, similar to massage. There are also specific stretches that target the obturator internus muscle. The first step to treating this muscle is identifying that it is a source of pain. Sometimes, this means ruling out other muscles, such as the hamstrings, as causative factors. If you feel your hamstrings or obturator internus muscles may be contributing to your posterior thigh pain and our suggestions for exercise are not helping, consider an evaluation by a physical therapist to receive an accurate diagnosis and specific exercises.

Neural tension in the sciatic nerve is another common factor in posterior thigh pain. Nerves move about seven millimeters in each direction. They need movement, blood flow, and space in order to stay healthy. Over time, the sciatic nerve (or any other nerve) can lose its ability to slide and glide as the leg moves because of muscle or fascial tightness, or trauma or injury to the area, or to the areas above and below it.

Neural tension may feel like sharp pain. It may also feel like a toothache in the leg, or you may experience numbness or tingling. Specific exercises that address neural mobility can improve the movement, blood flow, and space around a nerve. However, knowing which exercises to do and how many to do can be tricky. Doing too many neural mobility exercises, or being too aggressive, could cause your symptoms could flare up. Nerves are more sensitive than muscles, so in this case more is not better. We recommend seeing a physical therapist who can accurately diagnose sciatic neural tension to receive the appropriate exercises and instruction on how to progress with the exercises as needed.

Running form might be contributing to your symptoms, as well. If you are landing on your heel with your foot too far from your body or bending forward from your hips, this could result in increased stress on the back, nervous system, and hamstring. Some suggestions to improve your running form are to increase your cadence by five percent, or to make sure you are landing with your foot under your center of mass, with less heel strike and more weight on your midfoot as it hits the ground.

PLANTAR FACSIOSIS

Plantar fasciitis or fasciosis accounts for nearly 3.6 to seven percent of injuries in the general population, and eight percent of all running injuries[1,2]. Nearly one million Americans seek medical attention for plantar fasciitis a year, and approximately 40 percent of patients suffering from plantar fasciitis continue to have symptoms and pain two years after diagnosis[70].

Although the pathology of plantar fasciitis is not entirely understood, it is likely caused by microtears in the fascia on the plantar surface (bottom) of the foot. It is thought to be a progressive breakdown of collagen where the fascia inserts on the heel[71]. Some of these tissue changes, such as increased or decreased vascularity, fibrosis, fascial thickening, or even necrosis (dead tissue) can be seen on an ultrasound.

Plantar fasciitis is multifactorial. It is often attributed to overtraining and over-pronation of the foot. Other contributing factors include higher BMI, thicker heel pad[72], calf muscle tightness, and increased forces in the arch of the foot on landing or impact. As previously discussed, the postpartum runner has less stability in the foot and hips, has changing neuromuscular patterns, is carrying an increased amount of weight, and may have flatter, wider feet than she did prior to pregnancy.

Many people with plantar fasciits complain of pain in the morning, when walking barefoot, or after sitting for a long period of time. Many people describe their symptoms as sharp and painful in the heel, and pain can be exacerbated when walking on a hard surface. Runners will frequently say it is the worst during the first five to 10 minutes of a run and after they have stopped running[71].

PERIPHERAL NERVE ENTRAPMENT

Peripheral nerve entrapment is common during pregnancy or while postpartum, secondary to increased pregnancy swelling, biomechanical changes, or prolonged positioning during labor. Labor may compromise the nerves of the lumbar spine and sacrum and the peripheral nerves of the legs. The typical position of labor and delivery involves lying on your back, placing pressure through the pelvis and lower lumbar spine, with the hips positioned in extreme flexion and external rotation. This position, combined with the lengthening of the pelvic floor muscles through the pushing phase of labor, may place excessive tension on the lumbosacral plexus and lower limb peripheral nerves[65]. Additionally, increased compression and decreased blood flow to the perineum and peripheral nerves contribute to these injuries[39,65].

While nerve injuries are common in the lumbar spine and pelvis, as well, this chapter will focus on common nerve entrapments that occur in the lower extremities. Many of these injuries are present in all types of runners, but may be more likely in the postpartum population because of the tremendous change that occurs in the body during pregnancy. If you believe you have sustained a peripheral nerve injury, we recommend an evaluation by a physical therapist.

Peripheral nerves originate in the spine and pelvis, and often, it can be confusing to know exactly where the source of the symptoms lies. Searching for a physical therapist who specifically understands female runners and the challenges we face postpartum would be the best option; however, if that is not possible, most orthopedic and sports physical therapists should be able to treat these injuries. The physical therapist should take a thorough history of your previous running injuries and ask about your pregnancy and menstrual history. He or she should also assess your movement patterns and running gait, and should provide hands-on manual therapy in conjunction with exercise and neuromuscular re-education.

The most common nerve injury following labor and delivery is of the lateral femoral cutaneous nerve[39,65]. This is a nerve that is responsible for providing sensation to the front and side of the thigh. Injury to this nerve will result in burning, pain, and numbness in the anterolateral thigh. This injury typically resolves shortly after delivery, but may persist. In addition to injury during labor and delivery, pregnant women may also experience lateral femoral cutaneous nerve entrapment. Changes in pelvic positioning, increased intra-abdominal pressure, pressure from a growing uterus, the use of sacroiliac joint support belts, or prolonged hip flexion are all potential causes of symptoms[65].

The femoral nerve originates in the lumbar spine, descends into the abdomen and pelvis, and passes under the inguinal ligament into the anterior thigh. The femoral nerve is both motor and sensory in nature. It is responsible for the muscles that flex the hip and extend the knee, and for the sensation in the anterolateral thigh and the inner side of the leg and foot. Femoral nerve compression injuries typically occur during delivery. The femoral nerve typically has a poor blood supply, and compression from positioning in labor can further compromise the nerve. Excessive hip abduction and external rotation can cause increased stretch on the nerve[39].

These injuries can result in sensation loss in the anterolateral thigh, medial leg, and medial foot. In addition to sensory deficits, actions such as ascending or descending stairs, walking, and moving from sit to stand might be difficult because of muscular weakness. If these problems occur and do not resolve quickly, physical therapy will likely be needed[65].

The peroneal nerve provides sensation to the posterior/lateral aspect of the lower leg and knee joint. It also provides the input for movement to the anterior tibialis muscle and the peroneal muscles on the outside of the lower leg. These muscles control foot and ankle movement, and if this nerve is impaired, there may be consequences for gait.

Peroneal nerve injury occurs from excessive pressure during labor, when women are positioned in stirrups, when they have their knees hyperflexed, or when someone is holding onto their legs for a prolonged period of time. The pressure occurs just below the knee at the fibular head. Maintaining a prolonged squatting position, a common alternate laboring posture, may also aggravate this nerve[39]. Peroneal nerve damage may present as foot drop, weakness in the toes or feet, difficulty walking, or increased or decreased sensation on the top of the foot or outer part of the lower leg.

It is essential to recognize the signs and symptoms of running injuries as soon as possible and getting care for these injuries early on. The sooner you seek treatment, the sooner you will be out running again!

WHAT YOU NEED TO KNOW:

» The postpartum runner is a different runner than she previously was.

» The postural changes that occur during pregnancy may not go away postpartum.

» Overtraining can happen more easily to parents compared to runners who do not have children.

» Recognizing and correcting common postpartum postural strategies can be key to preventing running injuries.

11

The Postpartum Runner Is Different

Running is bliss for moms. Who cares if it is hot, humid, snowing, or raining outside? Sometimes, the refrain of "Mom, Mommy, Mama" repeated over and over, or straight-up crying, seems a little more tolerable after spending some time alone in the great outdoors. It's okay if your socks don't match, your shirt is on backward, or you are covered in snot, poop, your child's breakfast, or all of the above.

You are running.

If you are running without a child, know that we are all jealous. Enjoy every moment of silence or your adult conversations. No one will blame you if you sneak in one extra mile or stop and have a secret coffee break when you're done. The only question you need to ask yourself is, "How long can I run before the house burns down?"

This chapter will focus on some of the essentials postpartum runners need to know about their bodies, and what it means to be a postpartum runner.

After reading about the numerous changes to the body during the year of pregnancy, childbirth, and recovery, it should be clear that the postpartum runner will inevitably return to her sport a different runner than she was prior to childbirth. This is not to say she will be any worse or better off than before her child was born—simply different.

Not only has her body changed on this incredible journey, but her life circumstances have, as well. Priorities naturally shift as families begin to adjust to life with a baby. Incorporating new equipment, such as running strollers, can affect running mechanics. Overtraining can also happen more easily, as women put pressure on themselves to lose weight and get back to how they ran pre-pregnancy more quickly than their bodies will allow.

To effectively return to her sport, a woman should recognize these changes and know what to do about them.

COMMON POSTPARTUM STRATEGIES AND POSTURAL CHANGES

There is not one posture that is absolutely correct. Every woman and every body is different, and there is no way to fit all women into one box. Having a variety of postural strategies also helps women adapt to different movements and activities. While there is not a "perfect posture," some strategies are better than others when it comes to running.

After years of observing and studying runners, we have identified certain postural strategies as being common in postpartum women. In addition to these strategies, there are many other postural and biomechanical changes that occur in a woman's body postpartum.

Below, we will describe these specific strategies and postural changes, and how they impact the body's response to the physical stresses of running. Most of these strategies are normal postpartum, and may even resolve on their own. However, many women continue to use these strategies immediately postpartum and even years later. Our goal is to point out these changes: if you continue to notice them, do not ignore them, as they may play a role in several running injures down the road.

1. Butt Gripping

What is it?

This phenomenon is when the muscles of the posterior buttocks, such as the deep hip external rotators, the coccygeus muscle and/ or gluteal muscles become overworked. These muscles have a key role in the stability of the pelvic girdle and lower limbs[73].

What happens?

The butt-gripping strategy causes the pelvis to tilt posteriorly (backward), the lower lumbar spine to lose its normal curve and begin to flatten, the sacroiliac joints to compress, and the orientation of the pelvic inlet to become more vertical[73,74].

Why does it matter?

This is important because with these positional changes, the ability of the pelvis to manage intra-abdominal pressure (IAP) and support the pelvic organs may decrease. Continuing to stand or run with a butt-gripping strategy can ultimately affect the hip, spine, and pelvic floor muscles and lead to some of the problems previously discussed[74]. In running, each time you land on one leg, IAP increases, so having the most support possible is ideal. A butt-gripping strategy creates an imbalance in the muscles in the hips and pelvis, and is not an effective way to create adequate support with one-leg loading.

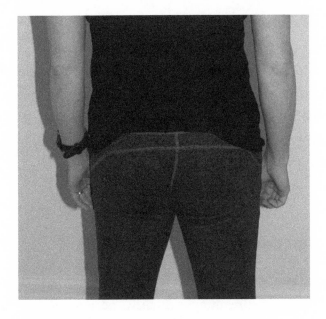

Example of what butt gripping looks like

2. Chest Gripping

What is it?

In this strategy, the external oblique muscles in the upper abdomen are overused, and the transverse abdominis in the lower abdominal wall is underutilized[73].

What happens?

Chest gripping creates tightness in the upper part of the abdominal wall near the rib cage, and less support in the lower abdominal wall. The lower abdomen can also become distended. This can cause the myofascia and internal organs to be under more load than what is ideal, leading to changes in function and structure over time[73].

Why does it matter?

Gripping in the abdomen can lead to chest breathing, and it also makes it difficult for the diaphragm to descend appropriately, ultimately impacting overall core stability. Additionally, the woman who employs this strategy may believe she is five pounds overweight, with a "mummy tummy." In reality, it is the distention of the abdomen, not adipose (fat) tissue, that can cause this appearance.

3. Dysfunctional Breathing Patterns

What are they?

Chest breathing: Breathing primarily occurs in the chest and cervical (neck) area of the body

Breath holding: Holding breath (usually an inhale) during exercise

Not fully exhaling: Inhaling, but shortening the exhale

Incomplete breath: Inability to breathe into the posterior (back) or lateral (sides) rib cage

What happens?

Diaphragmatic breathing is an important component of overall stability. How a person breathes affects her pelvic floor function, core stability, ventilation, and much more. Dysfunctional breathing patterns are common in the general public and are often seen in postpartum moms.

Why does it matter?

Learning how to breathe using your diaphragm is important in restoring functional trunk mechanics and core stability. In fact, addressing breathing is probably the most impactful and under-utilized exercise for postpartum women. See Chapter 12 for exercises that address this issue.

4. Posture

What is it?
Posture refers to how a person holds her body when sitting or standing.

What happens?
As discussed in previous chapters, posture changes dramatically during pregnancy. Butt gripping and chest gripping are two types of postural changes. However, other common compensations include sticking the chest out so that the rib cage is not over the pelvis, flaring the rib cage outward, increasing or decreasing the curvature of the spine, widening the pelvis, flattening of the feet, and changing the alignment of the lower extremities, such as the knees coming together. Once a woman has her baby, her posture doesn't automatically return to its former state.

Why does this matter?
Research suggests that many of these biomechanical changes resolve in six months. However, clinically, we have not seen this to be the case. Women one year, five years, ten years or more postpartum continue to demonstrate many of these postural neuromuscular patterns.

Accommodating the changes in the feet may require a woman to change the running shoes she previously wore. It may also be more important for her to begin strengthening her foot and arch to prepare for loading her foot during the running stride (see exercise in Chapter 12).

Prior to pregnancy, women are more likely than men to get knee pain because a woman's pelvis is naturally wider than a man's. With a further increase in the width of the pelvis due to pregnancy, lower extremity alignment and mechanics are further compromised. In turn, postpartum women become more prone to an increase in femoral internal rotation and knee valgus. Additionally, muscle firing patterns in the abdomen, hip, and lower-extremity change throughout pregnancy, as described earlier. Altering muscle actions may also predispose the postpartum woman to knee pain. Exercises to retrain and reactivate these muscles are very important (see exercise examples in Chapter 12).

5. Running-Specific Lower-Extremity Changes[26,32,75]

What are they? What happens?

Step length: decreases

Stride length: decreases

Cadence: decreases

Base of support: increases

Double support time (time on both legs between strides): increases

Why does it matter?

Lower extremity changes occur during pregnancy and remain postpartum. They affect how a woman runs and walks. They often resolve eight to 16 weeks postpartum, but may continue much longer in some women[32,33]. This should not discourage women from running, but it may be important to modify frequency and intensity of running.

Stress Is Stress

The body does not know how to differentiate between "good stress" and "bad stress." The stress new parents feel ("What the heck am I doing with this little human? How in the world am I responsible for him/her? What is a snot sucker, anyway?") is very real. The poor nutritional choices sometimes made and the lack of sleep that inevitably occurs only adds to the overall stress on the body. The life changes that occur postpartum impact how the body performs, making new parents vulnerable to overtraining.

Exercise is considered a "good" stress on the body in most circumstances. We know that exercising postpartum is beneficial. It can help reduce anxiety, improve sleep, improve mood, help with weight management, and create a sense of community. Training the body slowly and appropriately allows it to adapt to the stress placed upon it without breaking down. Some positive adaptions include:

- Increasing the strength of your muscles
- Increasing the size of your muscles
- Increasing your muscle power
- Decreasing your cortisol levels
- Improving your performance
- Developing stronger bones and ligaments

However, too much of a good thing can be devastating, especially when you are excited to return to running postpartum. Because of stress during training, the body can reach a tipping point, when tissue injury exceeds repair. This occurs when the body is no longer getting stronger from the stress of exercise and begins to break down. In order to avoid overtraining, make sure you are using a good return-to-run program (see Chapter 13 for a suitable program), and pay attention to all of the stressors that may be present in your life.

A great way to monitor your stress is to keep track of your heart rate variability (HRV). Heart rate variability is a measurement that looks at the variation of heartbeats in a specific time period. Looking at HRV allows you to see if there is any imbalance in your entire system, especially your autonomic nervous system. It is a noninvasive way to look at training holistically.

There are several free or inexpensive applications available on most smart phones to track HRV. Most of the programs are easy to use, take minimal commitment, and can tell you if it is a good day to train or not, based on the subjective and objective data you input into the HRV program.

Recognizing Overtraining

Recognizing the signs of overtraining is just as important as recognizing the cause. If you can identify the signs and symptoms of overtraining, you might catch yourself before an injury occurs and forces you off of the road completely. The signs of overtraining are not always what you might think, however.

Signs and symptoms of overtraining include:

- Decreased training pleasure
- Sleep disturbances
- Fatigue
- Vulnerability to respiratory infections
- Memory disturbances
- Decreased productivity at work
- Irritability
- Digestive disturbances
- Muscle soreness
- Loss of training desire
- Increased resting heart rate
- Injury
- Muscle atrophy
- Increased cortisol

Many of these signs and symptoms are also a function of being a new parent! However, they may also signal that it is time to adjust your training habits and listen to your body. It is better to take it slow than to be sidelined because of an injury. Again, this is where new technology, such as an HRV application, can be helpful in determining if you are pushing yourself too hard. Just because it is on the schedule doesn't always mean running is the smart choice. Remember: The schedule doesn't know if you slept the night before!

WHAT YOU NEED TO KNOW:

» Start wherever you are: You know your body better than anyone else, because you live in it every day.

» Some of the exercises below may seem boring, but they are necessary. Think about the finish line.

» If the exercises in the foundational, basic, or intermediate section are too difficult for you, do not progress to the advanced section, even if the exercises are more fun and you can "feel them more."

12

Preparing to Run

O ne of the most difficult parts of getting back to exercising after having a baby is knowing where to start. It may seem intuitive to just pick up where you left off before you became pregnant, or where you stopped exercising while pregnant.

Our first piece of advice: DO NOT DO THIS!

If you are not convinced that pregnancy and childbirth are times of tremendous physical and mental change and adaptation, go back and reread the previous sections of this book. Contrary to what you may see, read, or hear, bodies do not just return to the condition they were in prior to pregnancy or childbirth. Research shows that women who are active prior to and during pregnancy have an easier time resuming activity in the postpartum period, but success comes with respecting the changes the body has undergone and taking it one step at a time.

Our second piece of advice: GO AT YOUR OWN PACE!

You will get there. Every woman's body is different, and some women need more recovery time, slower progressions, and even professional help and advice. It is not a sprint to see who can get back to where they were the quickest, but rather a journey where you can enjoy each step, knowing that what awaits at the end is worth the process.

With that disclaimer in place, the upcoming pages will outline basic exercises to serve as a starting point in resuming exercise after pregnancy.

This is not meant to be a protocol, but rather a guide.

Similar to building a house, your body must have its foundation before it is ready to handle higher-level skills, such as running and other types of exercise. The foundation exercises are designed to build awareness of the deep core muscles (diaphragm, transversus abdominis, PFM, and multifidus/deep low back muscles), to start gentle pelvic movements, and to begin to strengthen the glutes, quads, hamstrings, foot, and shoulder/scapula muscles. These exercises also help minimize the risk of developing urinary incontinence and pelvic organ prolapse, both immediately postpartum and later on in life. Progressing slowly but consistently through these exercises will build awareness of the abdominal muscles and help recovery from diastasis recti (DRA).

Prior to the exercise instruction is a section discussing how to check for DRA. If you believe you have a DRA, please consult with a physical therapist who is well versed in postpartum recovery to ensure you are advancing and modifying exercises appropriately.

Also, any unresolved incontinence of bowel or bladder, pelvic or low back pain, pelvic pressure, or signs of prolapse are indications to follow up with a physical therapist before continuing to exercise. Please refer to the checklist in Chapter 5 to determine whether you may have pelvic floor dysfunction that needs to be treated.

The final piece of advice is this:
IF YOU THINK YOU NEED HELP, GET IT!

There are many qualified professionals who can help you stay on track or get back on track with your exercise program. If you are having pain that is not related to the pelvic floor, consult a physical therapist that is well versed in running mechanics and the treatment of runners. If you think you may have any type of pelvic floor dysfunction, consult a physical therapist that specializes in pelvic health right away. Here are two resources to help you find a physical therapist in your area:

1. Pelvic Guru/Global Pelvic Health Alliance at https://pelvicguru. com. This directory contains a number of pelvic health professionals, including doctors, physical therapists, fitness professionals, mental health professionals, doulas, nutritionists, and educators worldwide who specialize in pelvic health.

2. The Section on Women's Health of the American Physical Therapy Association at www.womenshealthapta.org. This is a member organization of physical therapists and physical therapy assistants who specialize in the area of pelvic health.

If you think you may be dealing with postpartum depression, consult a mental health professional. If you notice signs of medical emergency, including severe pain, vaginal bleeding that continues past six weeks postpartum or stops and starts again (not regular menstrual cycle bleeding), extreme fatigue, lightheadedness, or other signs that do not feel normal, call your OB/GYN right away. Our bodies are strong and can handle more load than we may believe, but they also tell us when to stop.

The best way to feel fit, and to return to an active lifestyle, is to progress at a comfortable pace, avoid persistent or new aches and pains, get adequate rest and nutrition, and have fun throughout the process.

Self-Check for Diastasis Recti

Lie on your back with your knees bent and your feet flat on the floor. Cross one arm so your hand touches your opposite shoulder. Place your other hand perpendicular to your belly button, with your middle finger just above your belly button. Curl up your head and shoulders. Measure if there is a split in your abdomen. If so:

How many finger widths apart is the split?

How deep is the split (measure by knuckles)?

Return to the starting position and rest.

Check again, this time moving your hand about two inches above your belly button, and then again about two inches below your belly button. Sometimes, the split is only in one part of the abdomen, so it is important to check the entire length of the muscle, not just one location.

Repeat the same curl-up exercise; however, prior to curling up, perform one preparatory breath. Inhale, and allow your ribs, chest, and belly to expand. Exhale so your chest and ribs lower and your belly flattens. Activate the pelvic floor by imagining you are stopping the flow of urine (or see "Pelvic Floor Retraining" below).

Once the pelvic floor is engaged, curl up.

Did the depth or width of the split change? Is it wider? Deeper? Thinner? More shallow?

If your split is more than two finger widths apart, more than one knuckle deep, and/or it does not change on the second curl up, you may require help from a physical therapist or further assessment before continuing on with more abdominal exercises.

You will note that some of the exercises in this section are the same as those in the Exercises for Pregnant Runners chapter. This is because even if you have been doing the exercises we outlined in that chapter, you may need to repeat or continue them once your baby is born.

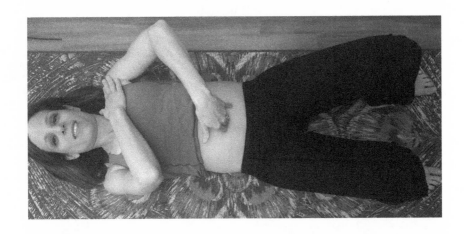

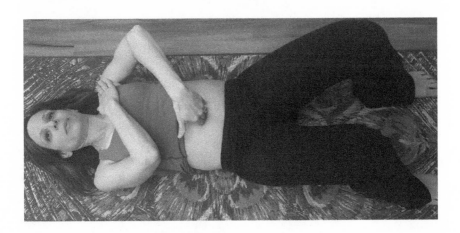

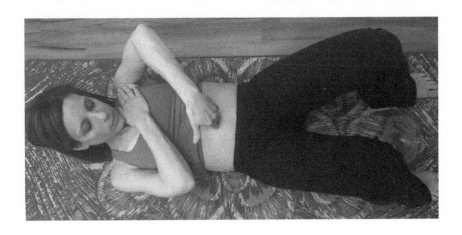

FOUNDATION EXERCISES

Practice these exercises as often as you can during weeks 1-6 postpartum, ideally daily. However, if you have been postpartum for longer (several weeks or years) and haven't done these exercises before please start them and do daily for 4-6 weeks. These exercises are foundational. If you haven't built a strong foundation you will be at higher risk for injuries.

1. Pelvic Clocks

The purpose of pelvic clocks is pelvic mobility. After pregnancy, women can lose mobility, general motor control and coordination because of the changes in muscle length and postural alignment that occur while pregnant. In general, doing pelvic mobility exercises just feels good. Additionally, spending some time with this exercise helps build awareness of the pelvis and the pelvic floor and helps to "awaken" the abdominal muscles.

Lie on your back with your knees bent and your feet flat on the floor. Imagine a clock placed faceup on top of your pelvis. Without moving your legs or back, tilt your pelvis toward your face (12:00) and toward your feet (6:00).

Starting at 12:00, move your pelvis in a circular motion in the clockwise direction. Imagine you are moving a hula hoop in a circle. The effort should come from your pelvis and not your hips or low back.

Repeat the circles in a counter-clockwise direction.

Repeat up to 10 times in each direction.

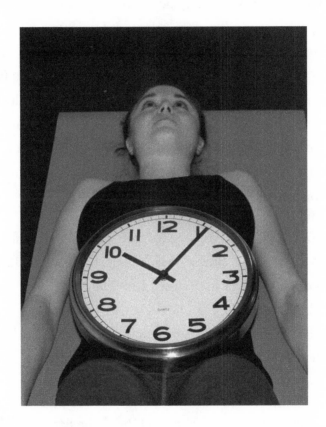

2. Finding Neutral Pelvis

Neutral pelvis is not one set position, but more of a range of positions that can vary for everyone. Having good pelvic alignment (along with the head, neck, shoulders, and spine) is important because the deep core muscles—abdominals, pelvic floor, diaphragm, and low back—work most efficiently when the pelvis is in a neutral alignment. Neutral pelvis alignment is the first step in building a strong foundation of core control, regardless of the position you choose to move or exercise. The following instructions outline how to find neutral pelvis while on your back and while in an all-fours position, but it is also helpful to be able to find neutral pelvis when sitting and standing.

Lie on your back with your knees bent and your feet flat on the floor. Perform pelvic clocks back and forth between 12:00 and 6:00. Find the position in between 12:00 and 6:00 that feels most comfortable. Your tailbone should be in contact with the floor. There will most likely be a small arch in your back. Your lower ribs should be touching the floor. You should not experience any pain.

Place the heel of your hand on the front of your pelvis, and your fingers on the pubic bone. Your hand should lie flat across the front of the pelvis. This is neutral pelvis.

Once you are in neutral pelvis, take a breath. You should be able to feel your ribs, abdomen, pelvis, and chest fill with air as you inhale.

As you exhale, you should feel the air in your abdomen release. In a neutral pelvis position, it is easier to activate the deep core muscles properly in order to take a deep breath.

Another good position in which to find neutral pelvis and to practice breathing is on all fours. Line up so your hands are under your shoulders, your knees are under your hips, and your neck is relaxed. Perform pelvic clocks in this position. Rock back and forth onto and off of your arms/shoulders to activate the muscles around your shoulder blades and upper back. Your back should not feel excessively arched or tucked. Breathing in this position should feel easy. This is neutral pelvis.

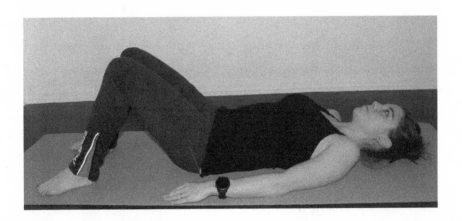

3. Diaphragmatic Breathing

Breathing is the hallmark of any good muscle training program. Women often substitute breath holding for optimal core muscle activation. The reality is that the diaphragm works with the abdominals and pelvic floor muscles to coordinate core control. Having nonoptimal breathing strategies, such as breath holding and/or bearing down with effort, can exacerbate pelvic floor dysfunction and diastasis recti. Good diaphragm function actually helps the pelvic floor contract properly. Ideally, the diaphragm, abdominals, and pelvic floor muscles should all work together.

Breathing is a great way to facilitate improvement in pelvic floor muscle activation, especially while muscles are healing from childbirth.

Start by lying down on your back, with your knees bent in a comfortable position. Find neutral pelvis. If you are not able to find neutral pelvis lying down, it is okay to try lying on your side, or sitting or standing. It can be more challenging to find neutral pelvis in these positions, but doing so is necessary to breathe well in all of these positions, as that is part of normal life function.

Take a deep breath in. As you inhale, focus on feeling your ribs expand and your belly and chest rise. At the same time, the pelvic floor muscles should be lengthening and relaxing. The diaphragm is a dome, and when it contracts, it flattens. As that occurs, the pelvic floor also moves inferiorly, but it is lengthening (opposite to what the diaphragm does). Coordinated movement of the ribs, chest, and abdomen is a sign of a good diaphragm contraction.

As you exhale, the opposite should occur: your diaphragm rises, the pelvic floor and abdominal muscles contract, and your ribs, belly, and chest move downward and inward.

Continuing this breathing pattern will not only help the pelvic floor muscles contract, but will also help them relax. For optimal muscle function, a full range of motion is important. In addition, breathing through the diaphragm helps bring oxygen to healing muscles and soft tissue and helps overall relaxation.

Practice breathing 10-15 full breaths.

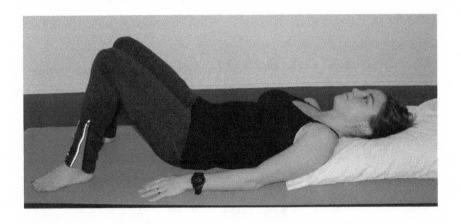

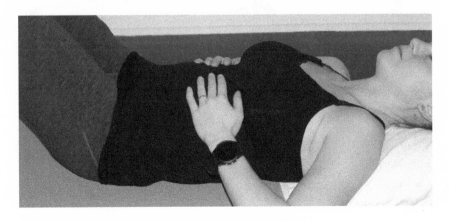

4. Pelvic Floor Retraining (Kegel Exercises)

As discussed earlier, pelvic floor dysfunction is associated with postnatal problems, such as urinary and fecal incontinence, and pelvic organ prolapse. Retraining the pelvic floor muscles has been shown to be an effective way to prevent, improve, and eliminate these symptoms. Remember, this exercise is just about building the foundation.

Once the pelvic floor muscles can contract, relax, and hold for several seconds, then the next step is coordinating the contraction of these muscles with those of the hip, trunk, and abs. The final step is to be able to contract the pelvic floor muscles while performing other movements, such as squatting, stepping, and jumping, in order to optimize everyday function and return to exercise without pain, leaking, or pressure in the pelvis.

Perform this exercise on your back or on your side with your knees bent. A good way to progress the exercise is to then try to perform the exercise on all fours in a neutral pelvis position or while sitting on a chair, in the car, or even on an exercise ball.

Perform one diaphragmatic breath (see exercise #3 above). Begin a second breath. As you exhale, imagine a kidney bean at the opening of your vagina. Gently squeeze and lift the kidney bean. Continue to breathe as you hold the contraction for up to 10 seconds. Relax completely before repeating.

If you cannot hold for 10 seconds, hold as long as you can for 10 repetitions. Work your way up to a 10-second hold. If this cue does not work for you, imagine you are trying to stop yourself from urinating. Lift the pelvic floor muscles up and in as you exhale to stop the flow of urine. Continue to breathe as you hold the contraction. Be aware of your hips, abdominals, and back. Keep them relaxed: avoiding tensing or tucking the glutes, pelvis, or inner thighs, and also avoid holding your breath.

Goal: 10-12 repetitions, holding each for 10 seconds.

Note: Do not perform this exercise while you are going to the bathroom.

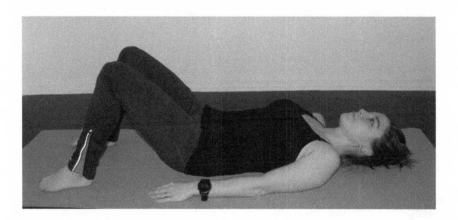

5. Curl Up

The curl up is a great way to initiate contraction of the rectus abdominis, which is the outer abdominal muscle. When you lift only your head and shoulders, the muscle can contract without placing too much load through the abdominal wall. By first breathing and contracting the pelvic floor muscles, and then lifting your head and shoulders, you can coordinate the deep core muscles with the contraction of the rectus abdominis.

Lie on your back with your knees bent in a neutral pelvis. Take one diaphragmatic breath to prepare.

On the next breath, as you exhale, activate the pelvic floor muscles. Curl up your head and shoulders so your shoulder blades lift off of the floor.

Reach your fingertips toward your toes. Your gaze should be between your knees and your belly button. Inhale as you hold this position.

As you exhale, lower to the floor.

Repeat 10 times.

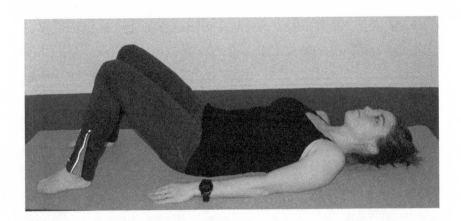

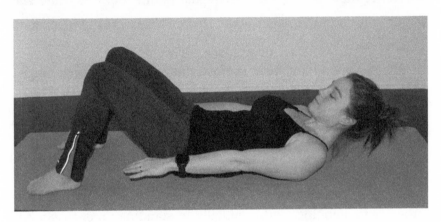

6. Intrinsic Foot Strength

Foot strength is often overlooked because its contribution to running is misunderstood. The arch of the foot has been described as "the core of the foot." When the arch collapses under the weight of the body, there is a risk for increased pronation, internal rotation of the leg, knee valgus, and hip drop. As described in previous chapters, pronation, internal rotation, knee valgus, and hip drop have been correlated with various lower-extremity running injuries.

The foot is the first part of the body to touch the ground when we stand, walk, or run. During pregnancy, the foot gets wider and larger to support the weight above. When a runner has a weak foot, balance and single-leg strength may be sacrificed.

Therefore, building intrinsic foot strength may improve single-leg strength and control. Running is essentially a single-leg sport. At any given moment in the gait cycle, the runner has one foot on the ground in stance phase, while the other leg moves through the swing phase.

Begin these exercises sitting in a chair. As they become easy, progress to standing, and eventually to standing on *one* leg while performing them.

Toe yoga:

Begin by sitting in a chair. Lift and spread your toes up and as high as you can without lifting the ball of your foot. All of your toes should spread.

Once you can do this, attempt to only lift the big toe.

Relax your toes.

Repeat 10-12 times, holding for five seconds each time.

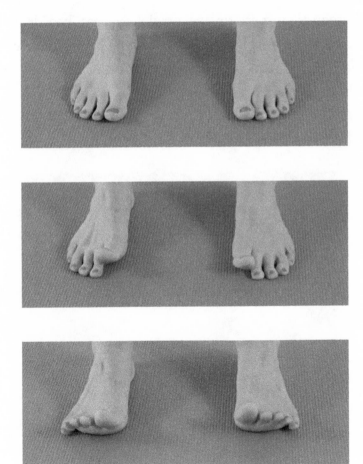

Arch domers/short-foot exercise:

Sit in a chair with your feet flat on the ground. Begin with your foot turned out.

Increase the height of the arch by actively attempting to lift the arch and pull the ball of your foot toward the heel without flexing or moving the toes. While maintaining the contraction, slide the affected foot across the floor to a neutral position. Return to the start position, and repeat.

As a progression, perform the previously described floor wipe maneuver. Upon reaching a neutral position, lift the inside of your foot off of the ground while maintaining contact with the ground with the outside of your foot.

Repeat 10-12 times.

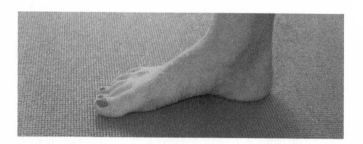

7. Check Your Standing Posture

Posture is an important building block for proper breathing strategies and for running form. There is no "perfect posture." However, there *is* an ideal setup when it comes to running. Using the "ideal running posture" helps the core muscles work more efficiently to support the lumbar spine, hips, and knees, and it also improves breathing mechanics with running.

Before starting to run, you should be able to find pelvic neutral in standing and learn a good breathing strategy. The first three foundational exercises are designed help you to find pelvic neutral and learn to breathe properly lying on your back. Once you are comfortable doing these exercises, try to repeat them in the standing position by using the following guidelines:

To check your posture, stand up with a mirror nearby.
First, notice where the weight falls on your feet.

Do you mostly feel it in the toes? Heels? Middle of the foot?

Once you notice where the weight is in your feet, take a deep breath. Do you feel like you can take a deep breath? Do you feel your breath more in your chest? Your back? Your belly?

Then, adjust your weight so that it is directly over the middle of your foot.

Take another breath. Did your breath change? Did it feel more full? More shallow? Different? Better? Worse?

Most women tend to stand with their weight in the back of their heels, with their buttocks tucked under and the rib cage flared to the front. Shifting your weight slightly forward so that it is on the midfoot will help to change the alignment of the rib cage and allow you to breathe more easily.

Second, are you leaning backward or forward from the hips? Are you tucking your butt under, or gripping tight in your abdominal muscles and holding your breath? You should feel generally relaxed in the torso, and like you can take a full breath.

Ideally, the rib cage should be stacked over your pelvis to assure the best breathing and deep core stability possible. Don't hold your breath or tighten your abdominal wall. Watch that you are not tucking your butt underneath you. As discussed in Chapter 11, these changes will impact how your body supports you while you exercise and run.

BASIC EXERCISES

Once you have mastered the foundation exercises, the next step is to move on to basic spinal mobility and abdominal and hip strengthening. The goal is to coordinate breathing and pelvic floor muscle contraction with different movements. The transverse abdominis is part of the deep core, and the obliques, rectus abdominis, and glutes play supporting roles in spinal stability and motor control. They also help to maintain intra-abdominal pressure with higher-level activities, such as jumping, running, cutting, and other types of high-impact exercise.

Practice these exercises as often as you can once you have mastered the foundational exercises, ideally daily but at least 4-6 times per week.

1. Bridging

One mistake many women make when addressing core and hip strength is to stiffen the spine and overbrace. Bracing is important in certain situations, such as when lifting heavy weights and doing power moves. However, for most exercises, the deep core muscle team works best when there is less stiffness and some movement.

Bridging is a great introductory exercise to coordinate pelvic and spinal mobility with core and hip work. It also brings the hips higher than the shoulders, which is helpful initially to address pelvic organ prolapse (POP), or the sensation of pressure or heaviness in the vagina.

Lie on your back with your knees bent and your feet flat on the floor. Find your neutral pelvis. As you exhale, activate the pelvic floor, feeling the abdominals flatten as they also engage. Begin to tip your pelvis toward 12:00, and slowly roll up, one vertebra at a time. Keep equal weight on both legs, and keep the abdominal muscles and pelvic floor working.

Take another breath, and as you exhale, roll down one vertebra at a time.

Repeat 10-15 times.

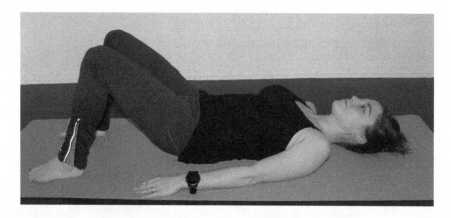

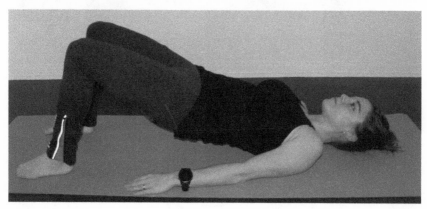

2. Roll Downs

The roll down is a modified Pilates exercise. It incorporates deep core muscle control with abdominal strengthening and spinal mobility. It is progressive in nature. Only roll down as far as you can get back up without having to brace, hold your breath and bear down, or feel like your abs are pushing outward. A partial roll down is safe with DRA, as long as the bulging or doming does not get worse.

Sit on the floor with your knees bent in front of you and your feet flat on the floor. Place your hands behind your thighs, and keep your elbows wide.

Take one complete breath to prepare. On the second breath, activate the pelvic floor as you exhale, and begin to roll down, one vertebra at a time.

Go as far as you can control the movement on both the rolls down *and* up, with the goal being to lie flat on your back at the end of the roll down.

On the next exhale, activate the pelvic floor, and begin to roll up to the seated position, starting by flexing your head and neck and using your hands behind your thighs for support and assistance. Do not hold your breath through any part of the range of motion.

To add a challenge, hold your hands straight out in front of you instead of grasping them behind your thighs.

Repeat five to 10 times.

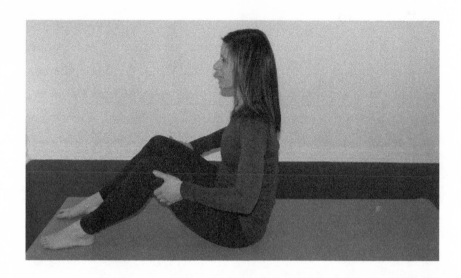

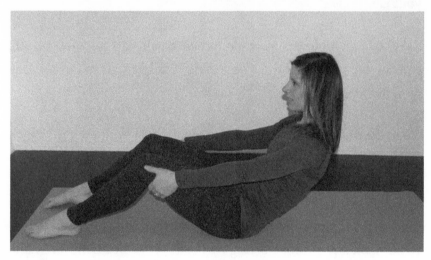

Rolldown, Stage One

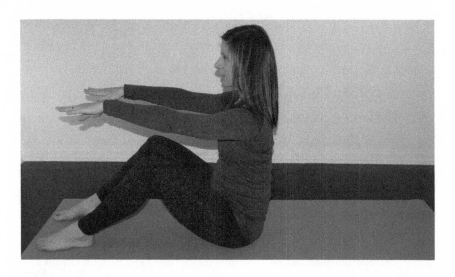

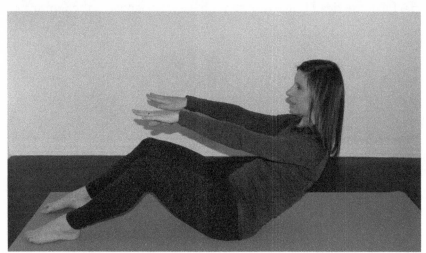

Rolldown, Stage Two

3. Dead Bug/Femur Arc

The dead bug is a simple but effective exercise to start to retrain the lower abdominal muscles. It also serves to coordinate breathing, as well as pelvic floor and abdominal contraction, while moving the legs. The key to success with this exercise is to use the diaphragm and pelvic floor muscles to help the abdominals draw in. To get the deep core muscles working efficiently, focus on coordinating breathing with pelvic floor muscle activation, and allow the abs to join in as they can. Overemphasis on drawing in, navel to spine, and tightening the core can exacerbate bracing and doming and have the opposite effect on healing of the abs/DRA. Once you can perform the dead bug exercise with ease, progress to the femur arc, which is more challenging.

Lie on your back in neutral pelvis with your knees bent. Take one diaphragmatic breath to prepare.

On the next breath, as you exhale, activate the pelvic floor muscles. As you do so, begin to lift the right leg so that it is at a 90-degree angle at your hip and knee. You should be able to feel tension across your lower abdomen without bulging, and your pelvis should remain in a neutral position. If you notice the abs are bulging, try to repeat the exercise, but only lift the foot minimally (two to three inches) off of the floor.

As you inhale, lower your leg to the start position. On the next exhale, repeat the sequence, this time lifting your left leg.

Repeat 10 times with each leg.

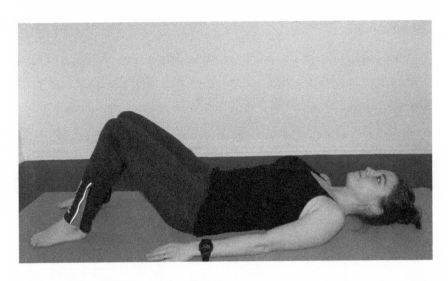

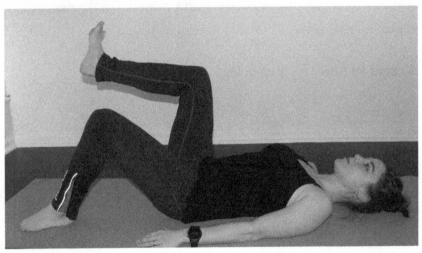

To advance:

Begin by lying on your back in neutral pelvis. Your hips and knees will be bent to 90 degrees, so your feet are off of the floor and your shins are parallel with the floor. Take one preparatory breath.

On the next breath, as you exhale, activate the pelvic floor muscles. As you do so, begin to lower your right leg toward the floor so that your toes tap the floor. You should be able to feel tension across your lower abdomen without bulging, and your pelvis should remain in a neutral position.

As you inhale, lift your leg to the start position. On the next exhale, repeat the sequence, this time lowering your left leg.

Repeat 10 times with each leg.

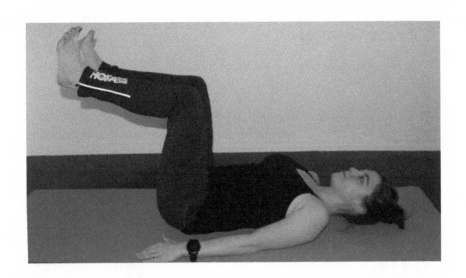

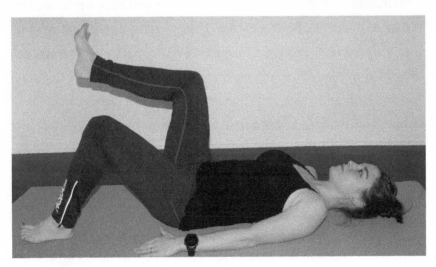

4. Pelvic Elevator

The pelvic elevator is an advanced pelvic floor retraining exercise. It is a way to work the pelvic floor muscles in isolation and teach the muscles to lengthen and shorten through a full range of motion. This is important because as you begin to add load (with weighted exercise or gravity) or impact (with running), the muscles need to be able to maintain control through the full range of motion.

Think of muscle like a trampoline: If it is too stiff when you land, it will not move, and you will not bounce back up. If it is too lax, it will drop all of the way down and not push you back up. The same is true of the pelvic floor muscles. They need to be stiff enough that they can support the pelvic organs with impact movements, but they also need to have enough flexibility to stretch and maintain tension with added load. They need to have the perfect balance of stiffness and mobility, and enough control to meet the demands of high-level activity.

Lie on your back with your knees bent in a neutral pelvis. Take one diaphragmatic breath to prepare.

On the next breath, as you exhale, activate the pelvic floor muscles. As you activate the muscles, imagine they are an elevator and that you are riding up from the ground floor to the fifth floor. Count to five through your exhale. On each count, raise up one floor.

On the next inhale, count to five, and let the pelvic floor muscles slowly lower down toward the ground floor. If you can, let the elevator drop down to the basement (below the start point). As you exhale, the elevator begins to move upward again. Adjust the timing of your breath so that you can inhale through a full lowering and exhale through a full lift.

Repeat 10 times through the full range of motion.

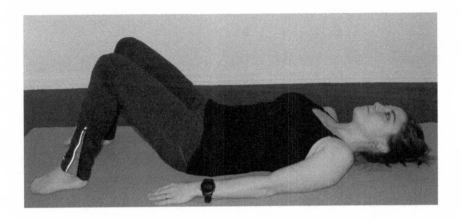

5. Pilates 100s

This is a classic Pilates mat exercise. The 100s exercise is more advanced than the dead bug exercise described previously. The emphasis is on breathing and core control. In the early stages of postnatal rehabilitation and return to exercise, it is best to perform a modified version of this exercise, advancing as your strength and endurance allow. Signs of a good, controlled contraction include continuing to breathe and not allowing the belly to "dome" or push out.

Stage 1:

Lie on your back in a neutral pelvis with your knees bent and your feet flat on the floor. Take one diaphragmatic breath to prepare.

On the next breath, as you exhale, activate the pelvic floor muscles. Curl up your head and shoulders so your shoulder blades lift off of the floor. Reach your fingertips toward your toes. Your gaze should be between your knees and your belly button.

Keep reaching with your arms as you inhale, and press toward the floor with the palms of your hands. Your arms should move in a beating motion, pressing toward the floor, with each beat equaling one count.

Inhale for five beats, and exhale for five beats.

Repeat for 10 full breaths.

Perform one set of 100 repetitions/beats.

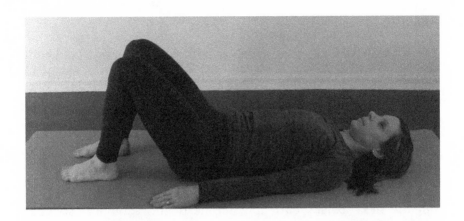

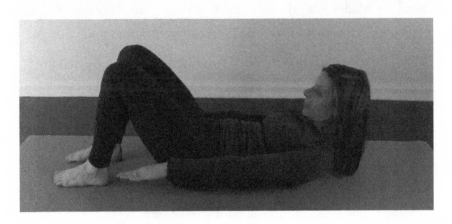

Stage 2:

Lie on your back in a neutral pelvis, with your knees bent and your feet flat on the floor. Take one diaphragmatic breath to prepare.

On the next breath, as you exhale, activate the pelvic floor muscles. Lift one leg at a time so that your hips and knees are bent at 90 degrees, with your shins parallel to the floor.

On the next exhale, curl up your head and shoulders so your shoulder blades lift off of the floor. Reach your fingertips toward your toes. Your gaze should be between your knees and your belly button.

Keep reaching with your arms as you inhale and press toward the floor with the palms of your hands. Your arms should move in a beating motion, pressing toward the floor, with each beat equaling one count.

Inhale for five beats, and exhale for five beats.

Repeat for 10 full breaths.

Perform one set of 100 repetitions/beats.

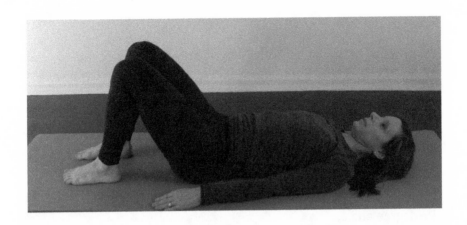

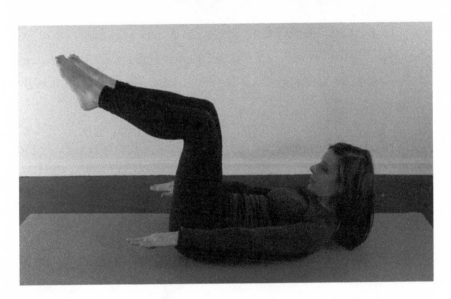

Stage 3:

Lie on your back in a neutral pelvis, with your knees bent and your feet flat on the floor. Take one diaphragmatic breath to prepare.

On the next breath, as you exhale, activate the pelvic floor muscles. Lift your legs so they are at a 90-degree bend, with your knees straight and the feet reaching toward the ceiling. For a greater challenge, move your feet away from your body at a 30- to 45-degree angle.

On the next exhale, curl up your head and shoulders so your shoulder blades lift off of the floor. Reach your fingertips toward your toes. Your gaze should be between your knees and your belly button.

Keep reaching with your arms as you inhale and press toward the floor with the palms of your hands. Your arms should move in a beating motion, pressing toward the floor, with each beat equaling one count.

Inhale for five beats, and exhale for five beats.

Repeat for 10 full breaths.

Perform one set of 100 repetitions/beats.

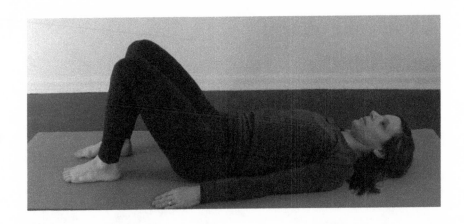

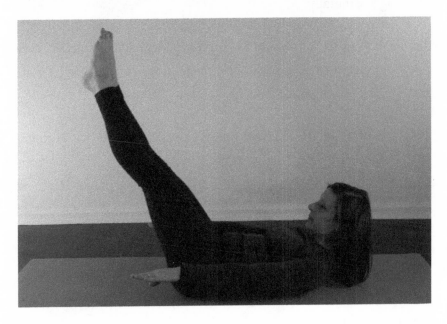

6. Side-Lying Leg Lifts

The side-lying position is a more challenging way to activate the deep core, maintain a neutral pelvis, and introduce movement of the limbs. In the leg lift, the hip muscles, namely the gluteus medius, work to lift the leg. The gluteus medius is responsible for control of the hips and pelvis when in the standing position. Retraining the hip muscles in the side-lying position is a good starting point for working up to standing exercises for the hips prior to returning to running postnatally.

Lie on one side. Your shoulders and hips should be stacked over each other and your body in a straight line. You can bend your bottom knee to improve balance.

Find a neutral pelvis position. Recall that in a neutral pelvis, if you place the heel of your hand on the front of the pelvis and your fingers on the pubic bone, your hand should lie flat across the front of the pelvis. Your back should not be arched. Your pelvis should not be tucked under with a flat back.

Take one breath to prepare. On the next exhale, activate the pelvic floor muscles, and lift the top leg about 12 inches. Your toes should point toward the front.

Inhale to lower your leg, and repeat on the next exhale. You should feel this on the outside of your hip.

For more of a challenge, prop up onto your forearm. In the propped position, your elbow should line up directly under your shoulder to minimize stress through the arm.

Repeat 10-20 times, and then switch sides.

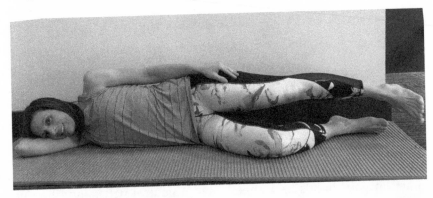

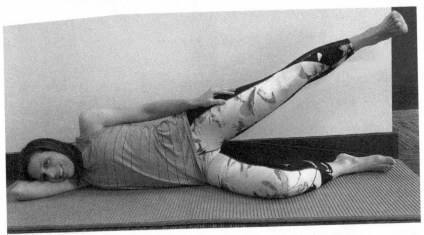

If you are not feeling this exercise on the outside of your hip, it might be too difficult. Try lying with the backside of your body against the wall. Your shoulders, bottom butt cheek, and top leg should all be touching the wall. Your bottom leg can be bent so that your foot is touching the wall. Take one breath to prepare. On the next exhale, activate the pelvic floor muscle, and push your top leg into the wall. Then, lift your leg about 12 inches. Your toes should point forward. Inhale to lower the leg.

Repeat 10-20 times, and then switch sides.

7. Quadruped Knee Lift

Quadruped, or hands-and-knees position, is a good way to address core control and coordinate arm and leg movements. This exercise is helpful because it activates the multifidi, the small muscles responsible for stabilizing the vertebrae in the back.

This exercise is more difficult than it may initially seem.

Start on your hands and knees. Find a neutral pelvis, and line up your shoulders over your hands and your hips over your knees. Keep your neck relaxed. Inhale to prepare.

As you exhale, activate the pelvic floor muscles. Lift one knee off of the floor, just high enough to slide a piece of paper under it without moving your spine or pelvis. Hold for five seconds, and return your knee to the ground.

Repeat with the opposite leg.

Perform three sets of five repetitions, alternating legs.

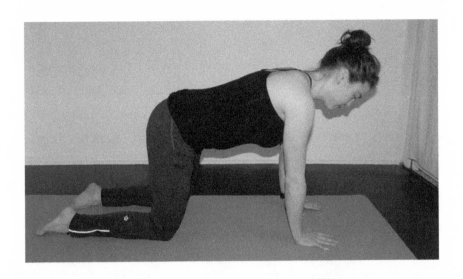

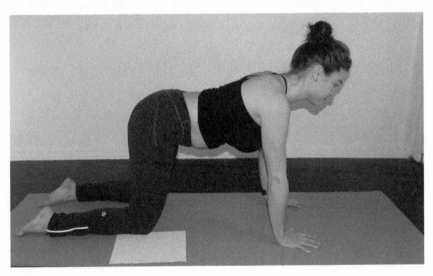

8. Assisted Squat

The squat is a basic standing exercise. While the motion is not complex and the assisted version does not add load, this exercise does involve moving against gravity. This can be a challenge for women who have symptoms of stress urinary incontinence or POP due to the weight of gravity placing downward pressure on the pelvic organs and urethra. By shortening the range of motion or using assistance, such as holding on to a door or strap, you can reduce the downward pressure on the pelvic floor muscles while retraining the muscles in the standing and squatting positions. Start with a smaller squat and increase the range of motion as you can, without experiencing pain, pressure, or leaking of urine.

Stand with your feet slightly wider than hip-width apart. Hold on to a door using both knobs, or use a sturdy table or chair that will not fall. Take one breath to prepare.

On the next exhale, activate the pelvic floor. Inhale as you lower your body toward the floor, being sure to hinge at the hips and maintain your weight on both your heels and toes, equally on the left and the right foot. Lower your body until your butt is just below your knees.

Exhale to engage the pelvic floor and glutes, and stand up. Use your arms as needed for assistance. If this exercise bothers your knees, limit the lowering to before the thighs are parallel to the floor. Keep the spine straight and the pelvis in a neutral position, with the chest lifted.

Repeat 10-20 times.

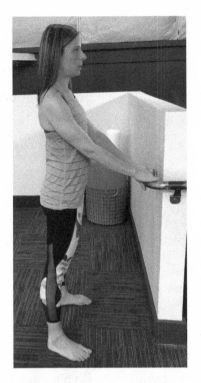

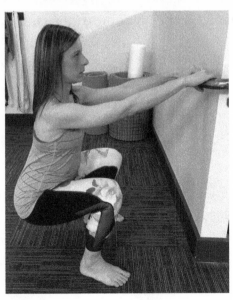

9. Single-Leg Balance

Running is a single-leg sport, and as such, it is important to have single-leg stability in order to run. Single-leg balance can seem simple, but there is actually a lot to pay attention to. Do these exercises in front of the mirror if possible, in bare feet, with good control of the arch of the foot. Refer back to the foot exercises if you are unable to maintain your arch in a single-leg position.

Stage 1:

Practice standing on one leg on a stable surface. Make sure you are maintaining good postural control in a pelvic neutral position, with your ribs stacked over your pelvis. Refer back to "standing posture" if you are unsure what good postural control in standing looks and feels like.

Do not tuck your butt under. Breathe. Keep your pelvis neutral. Try to maintain the arch of your foot. If you place your hands on your hips, you will notice if one hip is higher than the other; try to keep them level.

Hold this position for up to 30 seconds.

If you are losing your balance frequently, stand near a wall at first, and gradually progress away from the wall.

Spend three to five minutes on this exercise daily until it is too easy, and then progress as described below.

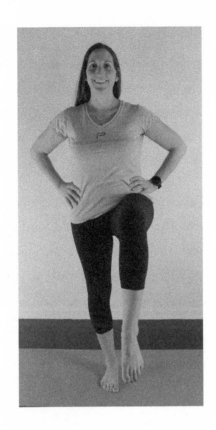

Stage 2:

Begin the single-leg balance with movement. Stand with balance as described above. Then, put your arms next to you, as if you were running with one arm slightly in front, with your fist at the level of your heart, and your other arm slightly back, with your fist at the level of your pocket.

Maintain your balance on one leg, and move the opposite leg through the air in an arc, like you would while running. Imagine your moving leg starting with triple flexion: your ankle, knee, and hip are all flexed (pulling your knee toward your chest).

Move your leg into triple extension, where your ankle, knee, and hip are all extended behind you.

Once this gets easy, begin swinging your arms, moving them from heart to pocket.

Spend three to five minutes on this exercise daily until it is too easy, then progress as described below.

Stage 3:

Add an unstable surface.

Repeat Stage 1 and then Stage 2 standing on a foam pad or another unstable surface, such as a pillow.

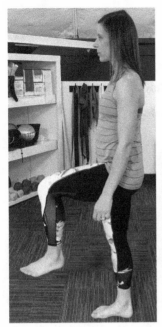
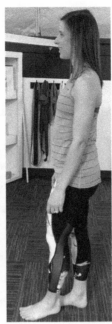
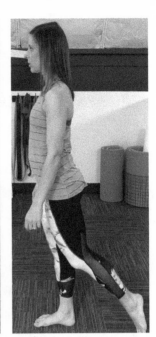

Stage 2 (above) / Stage 3 (below)

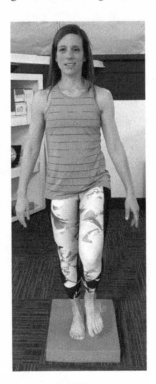

ADVANCED EXERCISES

Practice these exercises after you have mastered the fundamental and basic exercises. These exercises can be done anywhere from 4-6 times a week.

1. Back Bridge on Ball

The posterior chain, or back of the body, is incredibly important for running. The muscles in the posterior chain include the low back, lats, glutes, hamstrings, and posterior shoulder muscles. Bridging is a great exercise for working on the posterior chain. Using a ball under the legs adds instability and makes the exercise more advanced.

Lie on your back with your legs straight and your ankles on a ball. Take one breath to prepare.

On the next exhale, activate the pelvic floor muscles as you press your heels into the ball and lift your hips off of the ground by moving one vertebra at a time. As mentioned earlier, do not brace the abdominal muscles.

Take a breath at the top. Exhale, and lower yourself back to the ground one vertebra at a time.

Repeat 10-20 times.

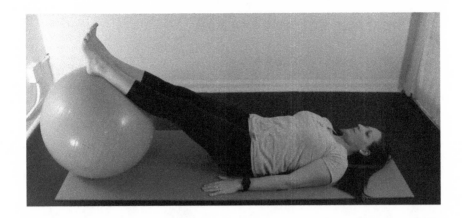

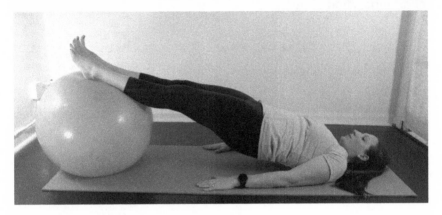

If you would like to increase the difficulty even further, you can try the following:

Prior to lifting your hips and back, lift your arms off of the ground, and cross them over your chest.

After lifting into the bridge position, try to lift one leg one to two inches off of the ball very slowly. Hold for five seconds. Return the leg to the ball, and repeat with the opposite leg before lowering to the ground.

2. Hamstring Curls on the Ball

Lie on your back with your legs straight and your ankles on a ball. Your arms should be flat on the floor with your elbows either straight or bent. Inhale to prepare.

Exhale, activate the pelvic floor muscles and lift your hips off of the ground so your legs and torso are in a straight line. Again, be sure you are breathing, and do not grip and overactivate your abdominals and glutes.

Use your legs to roll the ball toward your buttocks by bending your knees without lifting or lowering your hips.

Straighten your knees to roll the ball back to the starting position.

Repeat 10-20 times.

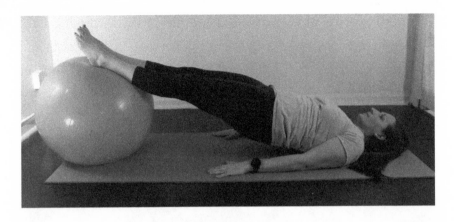

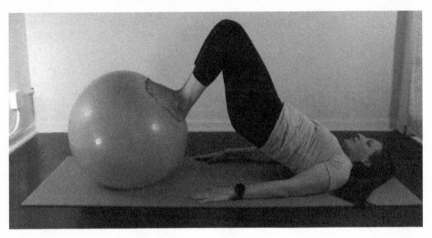

For a challenge, lift your elbows off of the ground.

A progression of this exercise is the single-leg hamstring curl: repeat the exercise as described, but lift one foot off of the ball, and use your other leg to roll the ball toward your buttocks, without lifting or lowering your hips.

Roll the ball back to the starting position by straightening your knee.

Repeat 10-20 times.

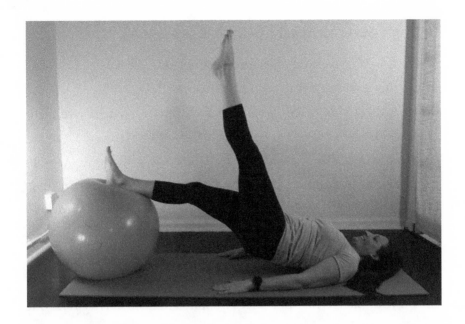

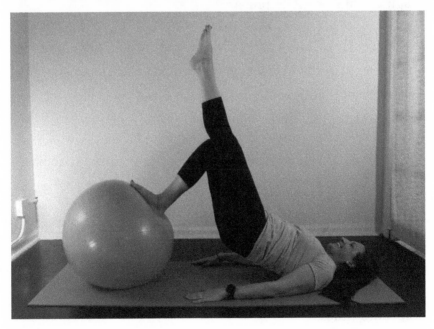

For a challenge, lift your elbows off of the ground.

3. Leg Lower and Lift (Abs Progression)

Leg lowering is an advanced abdominal exercise. It is appropriate to try this exercise when you have successfully mastered the roll down and 100s described above, at a minimum of stage two. This exercise also has progressions and regressions, as described below, so you can pick the version that feels best for your body. As with the previous abdominal exercises, be sure that you can continue breathing through the exercise, and do not allow the belly to "dome" or push out.

Stage 1:

Lie on your back with your knees bent in a neutral pelvis. Take one diaphragmatic breath to prepare.

On the next breath, as you exhale, activate the pelvic floor muscles. Lift one leg at a time so that your hips and knees are bent 90 degrees and your shins are parallel to the floor. Place your heels together, with your knees about shoulder-width apart.

Inhale as you lower your legs away from your torso, at about 45 degrees. As you exhale, return your legs to the starting position.

Keep your head on the floor, or for more of a challenge, curl up your head and shoulders. Place your hands behind your head and neck for more support.

Repeat 10 times.

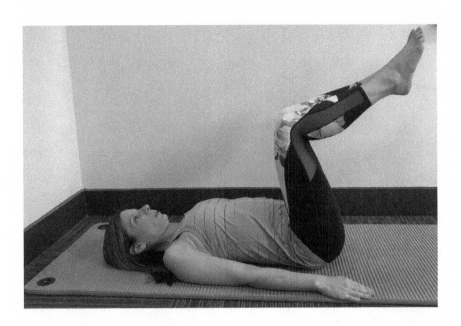

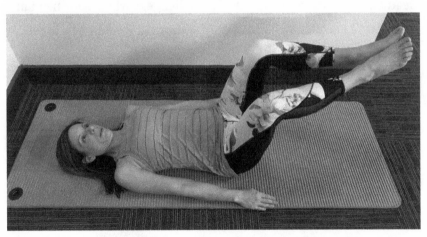

Stage 2:

Lie on your back with your knees bent in a neutral pelvis. Take one diaphragmatic breath to prepare.

On the next breath, as you exhale, activate the pelvic floor muscles. Lift one leg at a time so that your hips are at a 90-degree angle and your feet point toward the ceiling. Place your heels together and your knees about shoulder-width apart.

For more of a challenge, keep your legs together, parallel. Inhale as you lower your legs away from your torso, at about 45 degrees.

As you exhale, return your legs to the starting position. Keep your head on the floor, or for more of a challenge, curl up your head and shoulders. Place your hands behind your head and neck for more support.

Repeat 10 times.

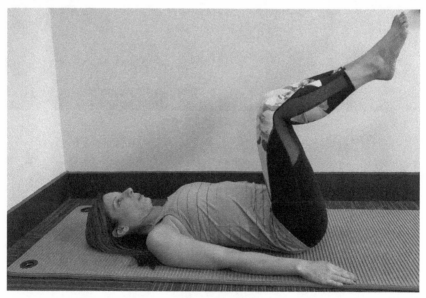

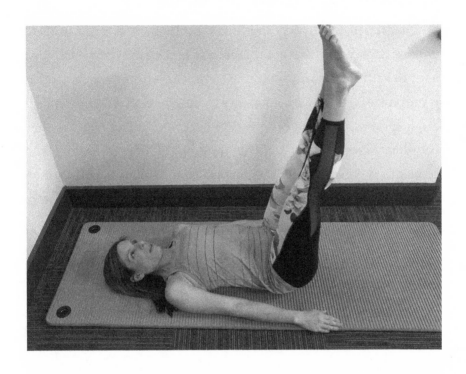

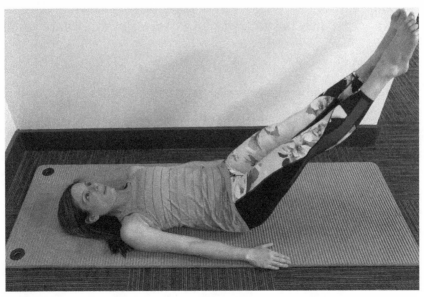

4. Quadruped Progression – Glutes

Quadruped, or hands-and-knees position, is a good way to address core control and coordinate arm and leg movements. Lifting a leg to activate the gluteal muscles also challenges core control, as it introduces a degree of instability to the exercise. These exercises are helpful as part of a progression back to running because they coordinate core and hip control. Try doing all of these exercises in sequence on one leg, and then switch to the opposite side. For an easier version, complete one exercise at a time on each leg before progressing to the next.

Start on your hands and knees. Find a neutral pelvis, lining up your shoulders over your hands and your hips over your knees. For each movement, your trunk should remain in a neutral position, with minimal rotation as the leg moves.

Hip Flexion/Extension:

Take a preparatory breath, and activate the pelvic floor muscles on the exhale.

On the next breath, inhale as you reach one leg behind you, parallel to the floor and no higher than your torso.

Exhale to bend the hip and knee, bringing the leg under you toward the chest.

Repeat 10 times.

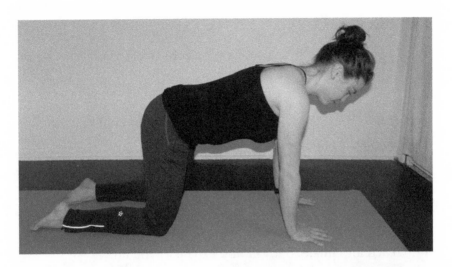

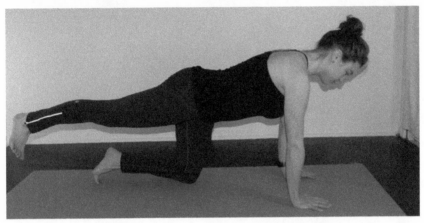

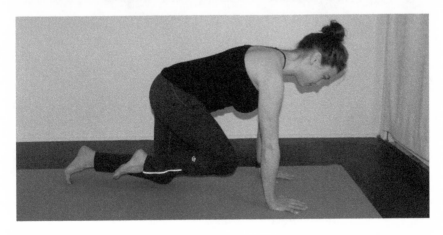

All-Fours Leg Lift:

Take a preparatory breath, and activate the pelvic floor muscles on the exhale.

On the next breath, inhale as you reach one leg behind you, keeping the foot on the ground.

Exhale as you lift the leg to the same height as your torso. Do not hyperextend.

With each lift, inhale to lower and exhale as you lift.

Repeat 10 times.

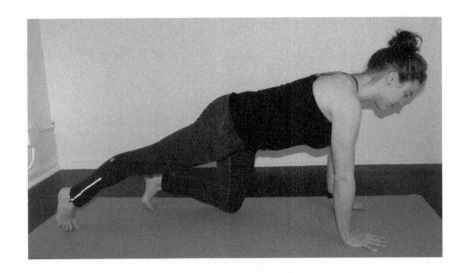

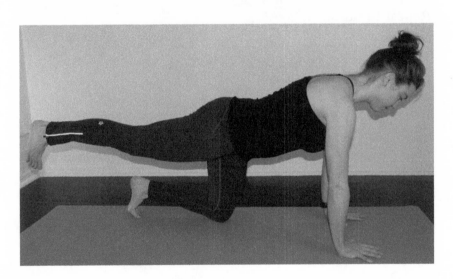

All-Fours Knee Flexion:

Take a preparatory breath, and activate the pelvic floor muscles on the exhale.

On the next breath, inhale as you reach one leg behind you, keeping your knee on the floor. Bend at the knee.

Exhale as you lift your left leg slightly higher than your torso. Keep the knee bent.

With each lift, inhale as you lower your leg, and exhale as you lift.

Repeat 10 times.

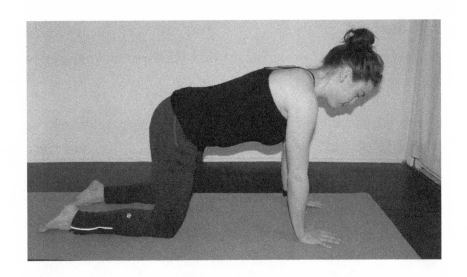

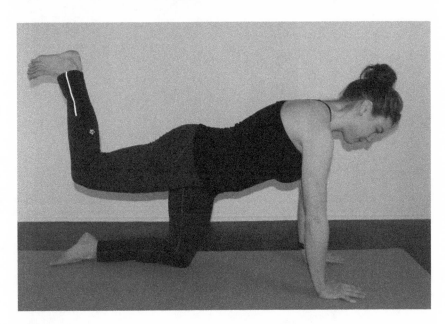

Fire Hydrant:

Take a preparatory breath, and activate the pelvic floor muscles on the exhale.

On the next breath, inhale as you bend one knee and lift your leg out to the side, to at least 30 but no more than 90 degrees. Keep your knee bent.

Exhale while you lower your leg.

Repeat 10 times.

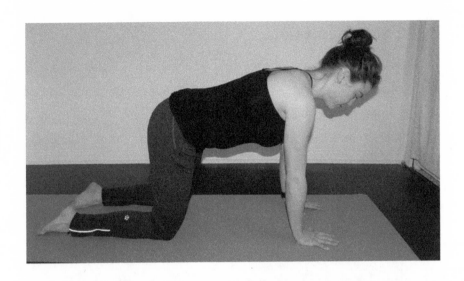

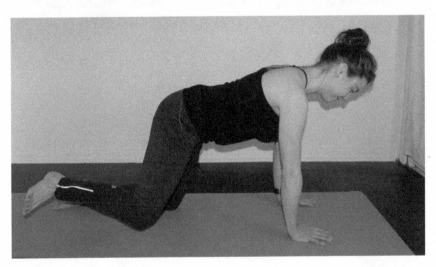

5. Plank Progressions

Plank exercises are more difficult because of the load the abdominal muscles and pelvic floor have to support in a lengthened and antigravity position. When performing plank exercises, it is important to maintain form, watching excessive arching of the back, lifting of the shoulders, and bracing and/or doming. In addition, you should be able to maintain your breathing pattern throughout the exercise, and you should experience no feelings of pressure in the pelvis. If you do feel pressure in the pelvis, the exercise may be too difficult for you at this time. The four exercises listed below are examples of plank progressions. If you can perform a plank or a side plank, feel free to add other variations of the plank exercise that you may know or like, as you are able.

Static Plank:

Begin in the all-fours position, maintaining a neutral pelvis. Inhale as you reach one leg behind you, keeping your foot on the floor.

Exhale to activate the pelvic floor muscles, and reach your other leg back to meet the extended leg. You should be in a plank position at this point.

Continue to breathe as you hold the plank for up to 30 seconds.

Rest. If this is difficult on your wrists, you may perform the plank on your forearms.

Repeat five times.

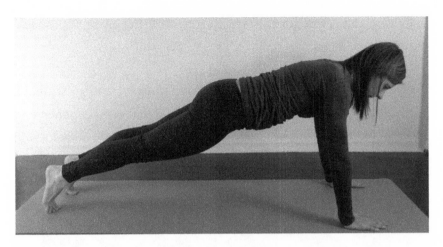

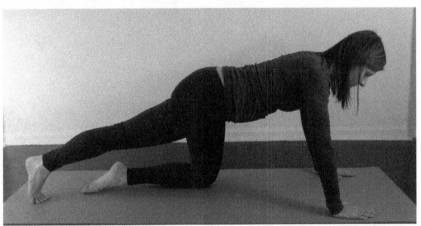

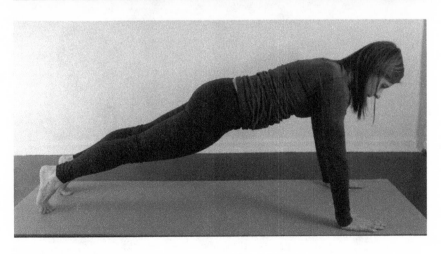

If a full plank is too difficult, try starting by lying on your stomach. Inhale to prepare.

As you exhale, activate the pelvic floor muscles and push up to a plank on your knees. You should maintain a neutral pelvis and continue to breathe as you hold the plank up to 30 seconds.

Repeat five times.

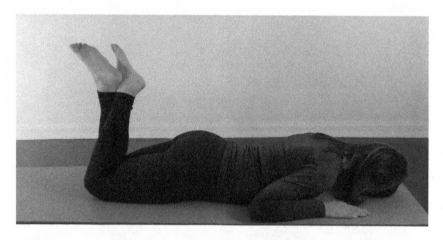

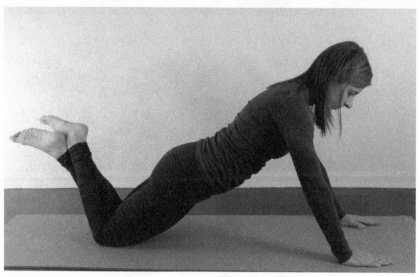

Plank Leg Lift:

Begin in the all-fours position, maintaining a neutral pelvis. Inhale as you reach one leg behind you, keeping your foot on the floor.

Exhale to activate the pelvic floor muscles, and reach the other leg back to meet the extended leg. You should be in a plank position at this point.

As you inhale, lift one leg six to 12 inches toward the ceiling, engaging the glute muscles in the buttocks. Maintain the plank position as you lift. Exhale while you lower your leg.

Repeat 10 times, and then switch legs.

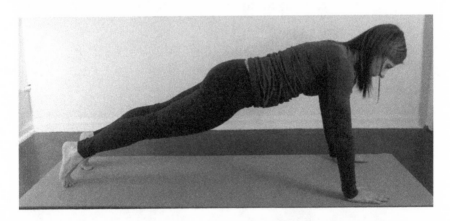

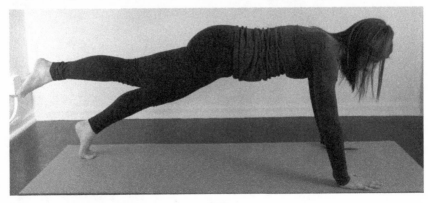

Mountain Climber:

Begin in the all-fours position, maintaining a neutral pelvis. Inhale as you reach one leg behind you, keeping your foot on the floor.

Exhale to activate the pelvic floor muscles, and reach your other leg back to meet the extended leg. You should be in a plank position at this point.

Inhale to lift one leg so it is parallel to your body.

Exhale to bend your knee, and pull it under your body, moving it toward your shoulder on the same side.

Inhale to return your leg to the starting position, and switch sides.

Exhale as the opposite knee pulls under your body.

Repeat 10 times, alternating sides.

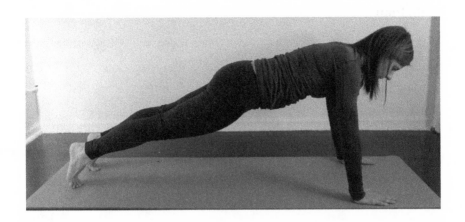

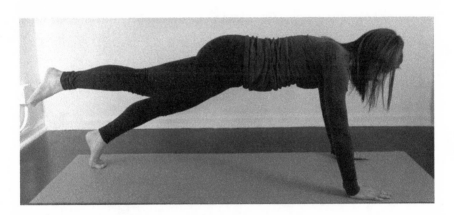

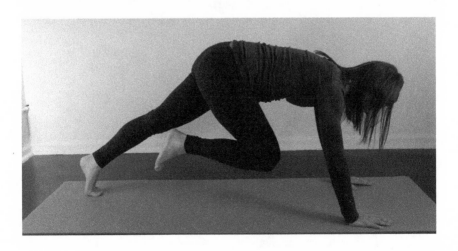

Side Plank:

Begin on your side, propped on your forearm, with your elbow under your shoulder and your hips and knees stacked. Your knees will be bent. Take one breath to prepare.

On the next exhale, activate the pelvic floor muscles. Without lifting your arm, imagine you are pulling the inner part of your support arm toward your torso, lift your ribs and then lift your hips from the floor. You will be in a plank, with your knees bent.

For more of a challenge, straighten your legs before lifting your hips. Continue to breathe as you hold the plank for up to 30 seconds.

Repeat five times, and switch sides.

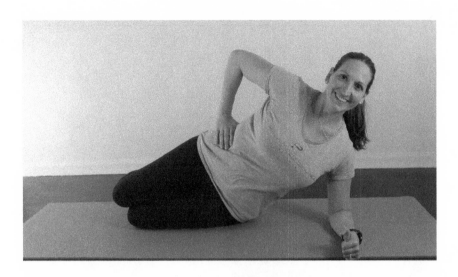

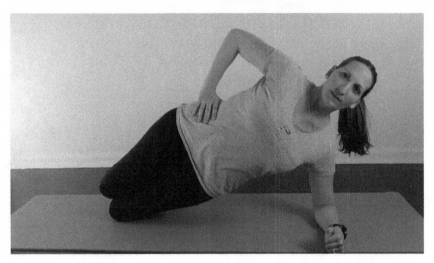

Side plank with knees bent

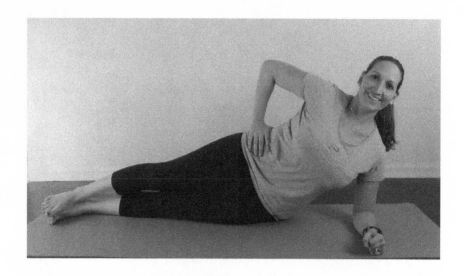

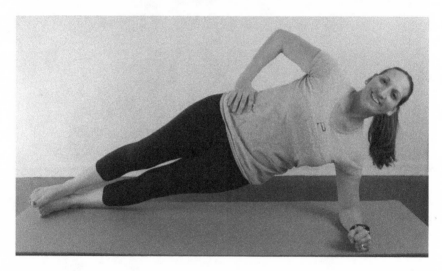

Side plank with straight legs

Side Plank Leg Lift:

Begin on your side, propped on your forearm, with your elbow under your shoulder and your hips and knees stacked. Your knees will be bent. Take one breath to prepare.

On the next exhale, activate the pelvic floor muscles. Without lifting your arm, imagine you are pulling the inner part of your support arm toward your torso; lift your ribs, and then lift your hips from the floor. You will be in a plank, with your knees bent.

Straighten your top leg.

Continue breathing as you lift your top leg, keeping it straight, until it is parallel with the floor. Be sure to maintain the plank position.

With each lift, inhale to lower, and exhale as you lift.

Repeat 10 times, and switch sides.

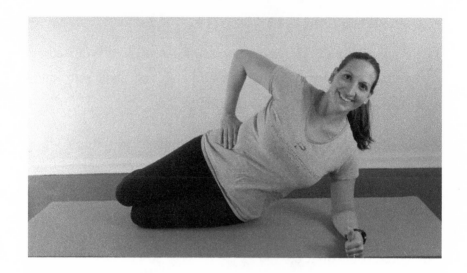

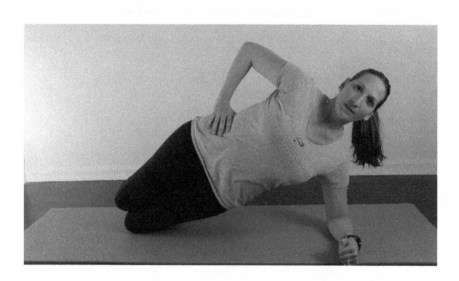

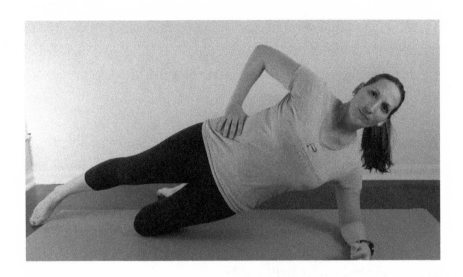

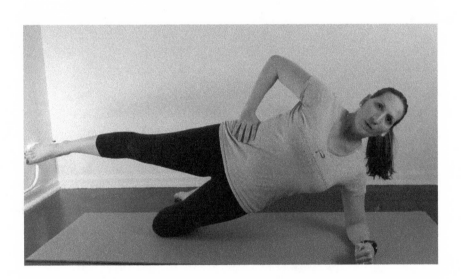

Once lifting and lowering your leg becomes easier, you can try to perform the arc motion: with your top leg lifted, flex it forward at the hip, keeping your knee and ankle in a flexed position, as well (triple flexion, as described above).

Maintaining the plank position, move your leg from the triple flexion position to the triple extension position of your hip, knee, and ankle, as described above.

This motion is similar to the movement of the leg with running.

Repeat 10 times, and switch sides.

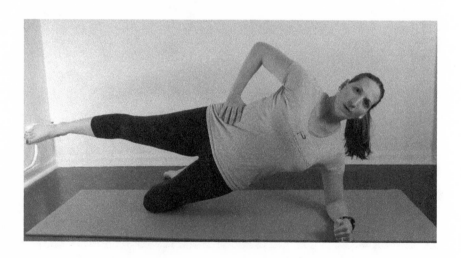

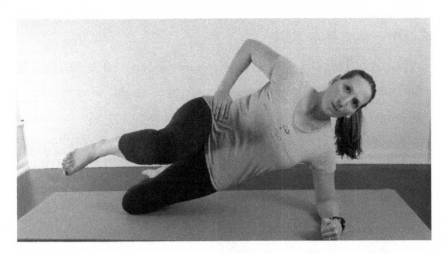

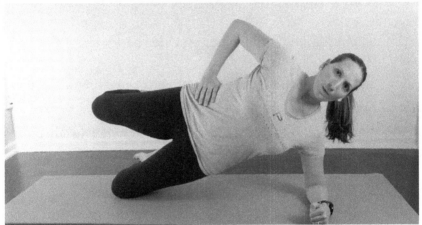

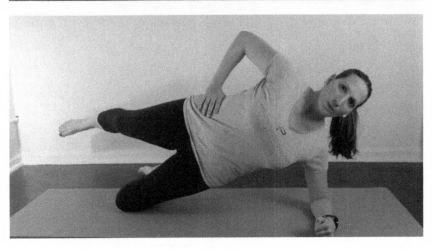

6. One-Leg Deadlift

The deadlift is an exercise that targets hip and core control, single-leg balance, and glute and hamstring strength, all of which are required for running. One-legged exercises pose a greater challenge to balance and allow you to work one side at a time, emphasizing the work of the gluteus medius to maintain lateral pelvic stability. Mastering this exercise is essential for you to return to running.

Stand with your feet hip-width apart. Take one preparatory breath. Activate the pelvic floor muscles on the exhale.

Stand on one leg, and extend your other leg backward.

Continue breathing as you bend forward, lowering your torso toward the floor, hinging at the hip. Your back should remain flat, and the heel and toes of your standing leg should be firmly on the floor.

Once your torso is parallel to the floor, engage the glutes and hamstrings to lift up to a standing position. Your hands may remain by your sides, or for an increased challenge, reach your arms in front of you.

For an additional challenge, try using a dumbbell or a kettlebell for added weight.

Repeat 10 times, and switch legs for two sets total.

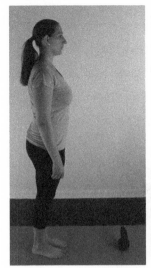
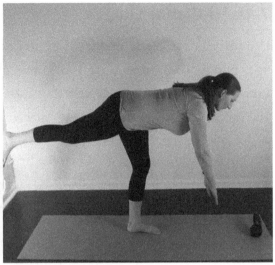
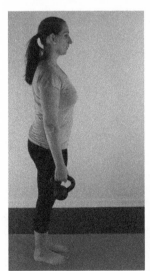
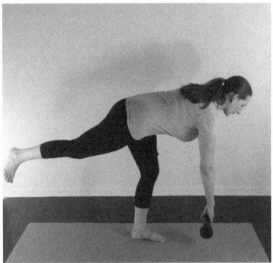

One-leg deadlift with and without added weight

7. Multi-Planar Lunges

This exercise offers another way to address single-leg balance and motor control, and to work the gluteus medius muscle. Practicing this exercise will help improve your single-leg strength and pelvic control, and may even improve your running form.

Do these lunges with one foot planted firmly on the ground and the other, your moving foot, on a towel or with a slider underneath the foot (they easy to find online, and usually inexpensive).

Posterior lateral lunges:

Stand with equal weight on both feet. Place the slider or towel under the ball of the moving foot. Maintain the integrity of the arch of the foot, and stability in the stance leg. Keep the hips and the knee of the stable leg pointing forward.

Slide the moving leg backward, placing it at a 45-degree angle from the standing leg, and turn the foot and the body toward the backward and outside of standing leg. Be sure to continue breathing throughout the exercise.

Return to the starting position.

Repeat three sets of five repetitions on each leg.

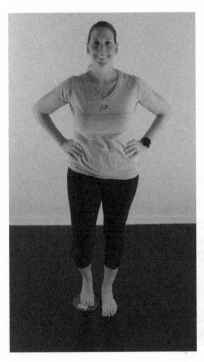 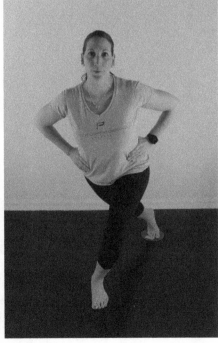

Lateral lunge:

Stand with equal weight on both feet. Place the slider or towel under the ball of the moving foot. Maintain the integrity of the arch of the foot, and stability in the stance leg. Keep the hips and the knee of the stable leg pointing forward.

Slide the moving leg to the side, keeping your kneecap over your second toe, and keep your hips pointing forward. Only slide your moving leg out to the side as far as you can comfortably control. Be sure to continue breathing throughout the exercise.

Return to the starting position.

Repeat three sets of five repetitions on each leg.

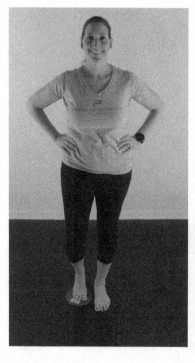
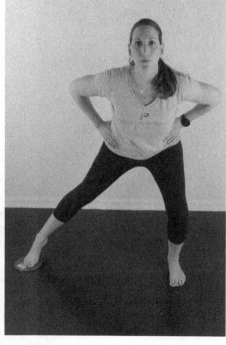

Backward lunge:

Stand with equal weight on both feet. Place the slider or towel under the ball of the moving foot. Maintain the integrity of the arch of the foot, and stability in the stance leg. Keep the hips and the knee of the stable leg pointing forward.

Slide the other leg back into a lunge position. Keep the support leg's heel planted on the ground. Be sure to continue breathing throughout the exercise.

Return to the starting position.

Repeat three sets of five repetitions on each leg.

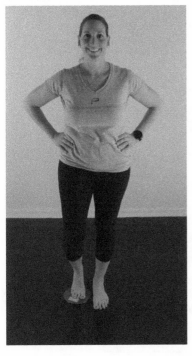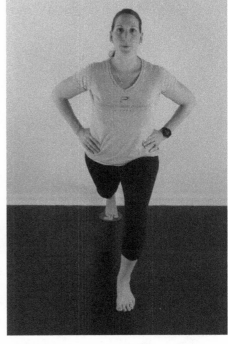

The exercises described above are meant to help guide you as you return to running. Yes, they may seem boring at times (we wish they weren't!); no, they are not nearly as fun as running (is anything?), but they are extremely important in helping you get back to running as easily and as injury free as possible.

As we mentioned previously, these exercises are not a protocol, but if you are unable to correctly perform them in the foundational and basic sections, it is not a good idea to attempt the advanced exercises. If you are having a difficult time progressing through the exercises and don't feel like you are doing them correctly, ask for help. Physical therapists that understand running and the postpartum athlete can be a great resource for you, and you may only need one or two visits.

It is always best to begin the foundational exercises prior to beginning a running program. The intermediate and advanced exercises can be done as you ramp up your running.

WHAT YOU NEED TO KNOW:

» Dynamic stretching prior to running is an ideal way to warm up.

» Running with a stroller can change your form: check below for tips.

» Follow the running progressions below, and do your best not to progress too quickly. It may seem tempting, but doing so will place you at a higher risk for injury.

13

Time to Run

The running plans detailed at the end of this chapter are meant to be a starting point. They are intended to guide women of all levels, from novice to elite. The first plan is designed for the beginning-to-novice runner. If you are less experienced, or perhaps did not run throughout your pregnancy, this plan is for you. The second plan is more aggressive and is appropriate for more experienced runners, or those who were able to continue running while pregnant.

While there is not a "one size fits all" when it comes to training programs, many women will be able to use these plans and successfully transition back to running without developing injuries. However, there are also many women who will benefit from seeking out a professional running coach to build a plan that is more individualized to their needs and running experience. Remember, you are not the same runner you were before pregnancy.

This is not to say that you are going to be better or worse. You are simply *different*.

Whether you are getting into running for the first time or returning to running, start by creating good habits. Make sure you are following a training plan to slowly ramp up your running volume (these plans will help). You should start each workout with a dynamic warm-up routine. Building hip, leg, back, and core strength will complement your running, regardless of whether you are a new, novice, or seasoned runner. The exercises in Chapter 12 are a good starting point to build strength. If you are unclear about how to achieve your objectives after going through this book, reach out to a professional for additional help.

GUIDELINES

The focus of this book thus far has been to help build you up to the point that you are ready to run after you have had a baby. It should be clear that we do *not* recommend starting back running without following the steps we have previously outlined, including working on the exercises in Chapter 12. Returning to running without a good foundation postpartum could set you up for injury, or if you are already injured, keep you on the sidelines much longer than you need to be. Our wish is for you to get back out there as quickly as possible, but in a safe way that minimizes your risk for pelvic floor dysfunction and other training injuries.

We recommend the following guidelines prior to beginning a running plan:

1. See a pelvic health physical therapist to evaluate your pelvic floor function, core control, and abdominal muscles for DRA.

2. If you have not seen a physical therapist, now is the time to check yourself for diastasis recti abdominis (separation of the abdominals). See Chapter 12.

3. Have your running form assessed by a physical therapist or running coach.

4. For the first four weeks of this program, run every other day for the time allotted. You may cross-train (elliptical, bike, swim) after your run, or on cross-training days.

5. Complete your breathing, abdominal, and posture exercises daily.

6. Complete a dynamic warm-up prior to your run.

7. Cool down by walking, foam rolling, or doing some of the muscle retraining exercises mentioned in Chapter 12.

8. You may feel a little discomfort as you return to running, but never run through pain. Ice as needed (no more than 10-12 minutes) to decrease any post-exercise soreness.

9. Repeat the same program as the prior week if you are extremely sore—make this about running healthily, not getting back to running ASAP.

10. *Do not* progress to the next week if you are hurting or limping. Consult your PT.

11. *Do not* progress faster than this program.

12. Most importantly, have fun, and enjoy the freedom of putting one foot in front of the other again!

DYNAMIC STRETCHING

Stretching takes extra time, and we know that time is everything when it comes to being a mom. It is tempting to skip a warm-up in favor of walking out the door and being off for your run. Starting a workout immediately after stepping out the door is not the best idea, though. There is mixed literature concerning stretching, but we do know there are benefits to adding five to eight minutes of dynamic stretching prior to beginning your workout.

Doing a dynamic warm-up prior to running, cutting, or sprinting will be helpful in improving metabolic factors that will positively affect your muscles, such as increased heart rate, blood flow to the muscle, and core temperature[76]. Other studies have found dynamic stretching to improve muscle compliance, nerve conduction, and possibly energy production[76,77]. Doing a dynamic warm-up is time well spent!

Dynamic stretching can include anything that targets some of the muscles used in running. Repeat each exercise for 10-20 seconds.

You can choose a combination of the suggested exercises below. We recommend choosing five to make up your dynamic warm-up routine:

- Walking on your heels
- Walking on your toes
- Side lunges
- Walking lunges
- Tipping over and touching your toes
- Walking forward while kicking your hamstring toward the opposite hand
- Squats
- Skipping

RUNNING WITH A STROLLER

Not every woman is going to run with her baby in a stroller. However, using a running stroller is beneficial, as it allows you to bring your baby with you while you exercise. There are certain implications of running with a stroller regarding running mechanics that you should be aware of, though.

This section offers technical and practical advice, should you choose to use a running stroller.

One of the first questions women ask is, "When can I put my baby in the running stroller?" This depends on which stroller you choose and what attachments you purchase. Some strollers can accommodate a car seat for younger children, and some cannot. Check the manual and specifications for your individual stroller.

We are not going to go into an evaluation of all of the various strollers here, as there are so many different running strollers available. Most of them you push, but there are some you can pull. Before you purchase a running stroller, test it. You do not want it to be too big, too tall, too short, or too heavy for you. Some running strollers have a fixed wheel in the front to improve performance, and some have a rotating wheel, which can make it easier to turn and maneuver the stroller. Comfort is key. Make sure your stroller fits you and your lifestyle.

Introducing an external load to push in front of you when you just had a baby is a big deal. We recommend running without a stroller initially so that you can work on your own running form as you transition back to running postpartum. The less stress added to the postpartum body while running, the better. If you have a partner that can run with you, it is ideal to have that person push the stroller initially. While this is not always possible, if you are fortunate enough to have a partner to help you, know that his or her mechanics will also be affected by running with a stroller, even if that person did not have a baby.

Running with a running stroller can affect the hip, pelvis, and trunk kinematics (motion)[78]. Holding onto the stroller in front of your body limits arm movement and restricts thoracic spine and trunk motion. Research has shown that running mechanics change when running with a stroller. These changes include decreased trunk rotation, a more rigid trunk, increased flexing forward at the hips, especially when going uphill, increased number of steps, reduced step length, the pelvis tending to tip forward, and typically less hip extension[78-80].

Unfortunately, many of these changes also correlate with increased lower back pain, increased pressure on the lower back facet joints, increased neural tension, lower extremity injuries, decreased gluteus muscle firing, and much more. This is not to say don't run with a stroller. Many times, the only way to stay on a consistent running schedule is to put your baby in a running stroller and take him or her with you. Be mindful of your posture and mechanics as you run with a stroller, however, especially if this is new to you. Below are some recommendations for pushing a running stroller as safely as possible.

Recommendation	Benefit
Lean from the ankles, not from the hips.	This helps maintain good running posture—rib cage over pelvis— in order to tap into the diaphragm-pelvic floor piston discussed in previous chapters.
Keep the stroller close.	Doing so prevents leaning forward from the hips, which impacts breathing and your core strength.
Push the stroller with one arm at a time, switching periodically. The arm that is swinging should move heart to pocket.	This will help improve thoracic spine motion and prevent overusing one side of the body.
Shorten your stride.	Shortening your stride improves gluteus muscle firing and will help you maintain good posture while running.

What Should I Pack in My Stroller?

Packing extra items as you head out with your baby for a run has nothing to do with body mechanics, posture, or breathing. This is simply a list from two moms who have learned the hard way how to be prepared for anything and everything that can happen while you are out on a run with your baby. After all, nobody wants to be caught out on a blissful run with a baby or toddler covered in poo!

First, it is important to know that many strollers have various attachments, such as rain covers, sun shields, snack trays, tire pumps, and water and key holders. These accessories will likely make it easier for you to run and get out of the house, no matter the weather, with everything you might need.

Here is the list of things we believe you shouldn't live without:

For babies:

- Rain/wind shield
- Extra diapers, wipes, and plastic bags for dirty diapers
- A lightweight, foldable changing pad
- A bottle or squeezable food pack
- A toy
- Blanket
- Sunscreen
- Water for you
- Nursing pads if you are breastfeeding
- Your phone

For toddlers:

- Rain/wind shield
- Extra underwear
- Wipes
- Water for both of you
- Sunscreen
- Toys or a book
- Snacks
- Your phone

Novice Running Program 1:

Purpose:

This running program is intended for individuals who have decided to run after having a baby, but who may not have run at all prior to pregnancy, *or* who have not run in more than one or two years. Remember, post-exercise soreness is normal, but pain is not. If you had a particularly difficult birth or you are not comfortable with the programs outlined, seek out a coach or physical therapist to help you.

Prior to starting this plan, walk at a comfortable pace two to three times per week for 15-20 minutes.

To download a copy of these charts, visit:
www.precisionpt.org/shop

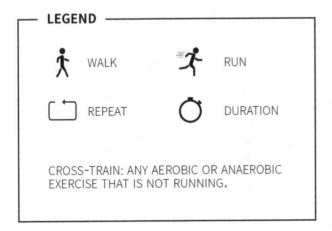

LEGEND

WALK   RUN

REPEAT   DURATION

CROSS-TRAIN: ANY AEROBIC OR ANAEROBIC EXERCISE THAT IS NOT RUNNING.

	WEEK 1	WEEK 2

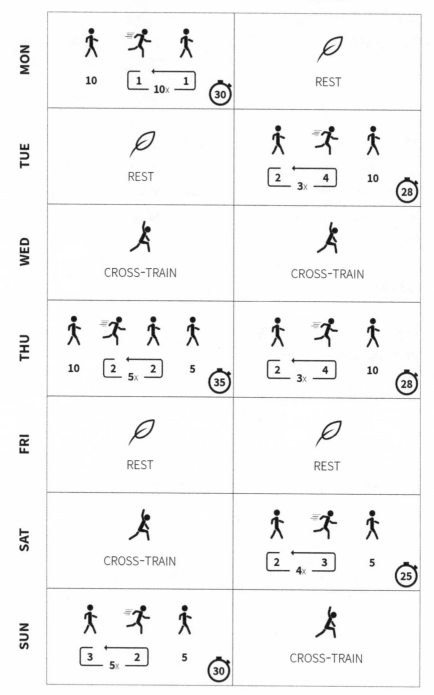

WEEK 3	WEEK 4	
Walk/Run: 2 ← 4 4x (24)	REST	MON
REST	Walk/Run: 2 ← 5 4x (28)	TUE
Walk/Run: 2 ← 5 4x (28)	CROSS-TRAIN	WED
CROSS-TRAIN	Walk/Run: 2 ← 6 4x (32)	THU
Walk/Run: 2 ← 4 4x (24)	REST	FRI
REST	Walk/Run: 2 ← 5 4x (28)	SAT
Walk/Run: 2 ← 5 4x (28)	CROSS-TRAIN **	SUN

** BEGIN PROGRAM 2 IN **WEEK 5**

Return to Running
Program 2:

Purpose:

This running program is intended for the woman who has had a baby in the last six months and was active during pregnancy. She may have run a little bit during pregnancy, but not consistently.

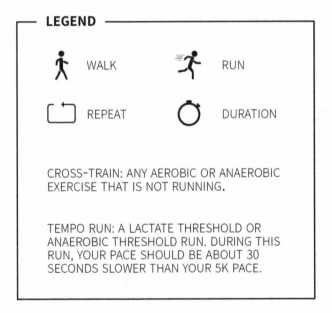

LEGEND

🚶 WALK   🏃 RUN

⟲ REPEAT   ⏱ DURATION

CROSS-TRAIN: ANY AEROBIC OR ANAEROBIC EXERCISE THAT IS NOT RUNNING.

TEMPO RUN: A LACTATE THRESHOLD OR ANAEROBIC THRESHOLD RUN. DURING THIS RUN, YOUR PACE SHOULD BE ABOUT 30 SECONDS SLOWER THAN YOUR 5K PACE.

	WEEK 1	WEEK 2
MON	🚶 🏃 🚶 🏃 10　5　5　5　⏱(25)	🏃 CROSS-TRAIN
TUE	🏃 CROSS-TRAIN	🚶 🏃 [2 ← 8]　3x　⏱(30)
WED	🏃 CROSS-TRAIN	🏃 CROSS-TRAIN
THU	🚶 🏃 [5 ← 5]　4x　⏱(40)	🚶 🏃 🚶 [2 ← 10]　3x　6　⏱(42)
FRI	🏃 CROSS-TRAIN	🏃 CROSS-TRAIN
SAT	🏃 CROSS-TRAIN	🚶 🏃 [2 ← 10]　3x　⏱(36)
SUN	🚶 🏃 [3 ← 7]　3x　⏱(30)	🏃 CROSS-TRAIN

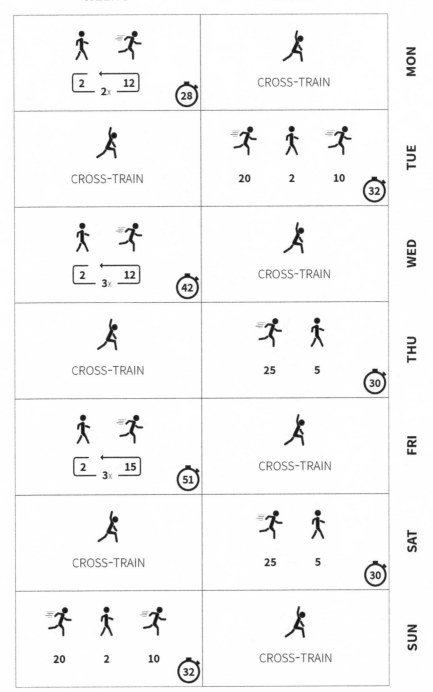

	WEEK 5	WEEK 6
MON	30 — 30	30 — 30
TUE	CROSS-TRAIN	CROSS-TRAIN OR REST
WED	30 — 30	30 — 30
THU	CROSS-TRAIN	35 — 35
FRI	25 — 25	CROSS-TRAIN OR REST
SAT	35 — 35	30 — 30
SUN	REST	CROSS-TRAIN OR REST

	WEEK 7	WEEK 8	
MON	40 · ⏱40	40 · ⏱40	
TUE	40 · ⏱40	CROSS-TRAIN OR REST	
WED	REST	30 · ⏱30	
THU	35 · ⏱35	30 · 5x 1 MIN "TEMPO" (APPROX 15K HM EFFORT) WITH 1 MIN EASY IN THE MIDDLE · ⏱30	
FRI	CROSS-TRAIN OR REST	CROSS-TRAIN OR REST	
SAT	30 · 5x 1 MIN "TEMPO" (APPROX 15K HM EFFORT) WITH 1 MIN EASY IN THE MIDDLE · ⏱30	50 · ⏱50	
SUN	CROSS-TRAIN OR REST	REST	

	WEEK 9	WEEK 10
MON	REST	REST
TUE	50 — 50	40 — 40
WED	30 — 5x 1 MIN "TEMPO" (APPROX 15K HM EFFORT) WITH 1 MIN EASY IN THE MIDDLE — 30	30 — 5x 1 MIN "TEMPO" (APPROX 15K HM EFFORT) WITH 1 MIN EASY IN THE MIDDLE — 30
THU	CROSS-TRAIN OR REST	CROSS-TRAIN OR REST
FRI	30 — 30	30 — 30
SAT	CROSS-TRAIN OR REST	30 OR CROSS-TRAIN
SUN	55 — 55	60 — 60

14

Go Out There and Kill the Hills

A ll of the tools are now at your feet. You've learned why our bodies do what they do during pregnancy, how they recover postpartum, and some of the things that can happen when you go back to running. We've dispelled some myths, and hopefully made you feel like you can safely get back out on the road or trails. We've given you information about pelvic floor dysfunction and what to do if you are experiencing any of these symptoms. You also have exercises to work through and detailed programs to get you started. We leave you with only two pieces of advice:

BE KIND TO YOURSELF!

Remember, recovery from pregnancy is a marathon. Sometimes, it feels like you will never see the finish line. Your body is healing. This can take several months, or even one to two years. If you have multiple children, it may take longer with each return from pregnancy. Your body is not the same as it was before pregnancy, so don't push it like it is. Respect the changes it has gone through, and the recovery period. You may continue to have ligament laxity. If you are breastfeeding, you may be at higher risk for stress fractures because the milk you are producing is taking the calcium from your bones. Recovery from pelvic organ prolapse and other pelvic floor dysfunction takes time. Like other muscle injuries, the pelvic floor muscles need time to heal and become strong again. If you ever have sharp pain with running or walking, or something just does not feel right, stop immediately and discuss it with your physical therapist or your doctor.

ENJOY THE JOURNEY!

We run because of how it makes us feel: strong, free from worry, and independent. Running is not just exercise, but a way of life. We understand that being a runner is part of who you are, because it is part of who *we* are. We have been in your shoes. Some days are joyous: perfect weather, a baby who sleeps through your run, the perfect stride, and a great workout mix to listen to. Other days we'd rather forget: cool and windy conditions, a child who can't be soothed, a diaper blowout two miles into your run, muscle soreness, or a stiff back. There will be ups and downs, and it's important to respect that. Just know that you have a tribe of women all around the world, who are working hard just like you, and that they have your back.

We've given you the good, the bad, and the ugly about running through pregnancy and what to expect postpartum. We've gotten super-technical, and we've offered some practical advice. We've shared our best mom experiences and our best knowledge as physical therapists. You have the tools and the information, and the support of many. Motherhood has so many joys, and showing your kids that you like to be strong and active is just one of them.

Now, go out there and kill the hills!

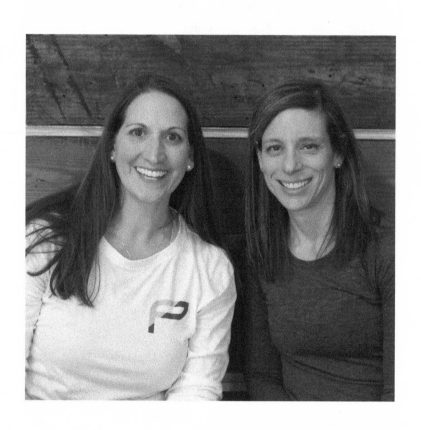

About the Authors

Dr. Kate Edwards PT, DPT, is a board-certified orthopaedic clinical specialist (OCS) and CEO/owner of Precision Performance & Physical Therapy in Atlanta, Georgia. Kate is an adjunct faculty member at Emory University School of Medicine in the department of physical therapy, where she teaches a course titled "The Endurance Athlete." She regularly contributes to research regarding runners, national publications, such as *Runner's World*, *Women's Running*, and *Triathlete* magazine, as well as mainstream media, such as CNN.

Her practice is a concierge-style physical therapy clinic that specializes in treating runners, triathletes, and complicated patients. As a runner and mother of a son, she is well versed in running during pregnancy and postpartum, and regularly helps female athletes transition from pregnancy back to endurance sports. She is a former triathlete and Boston Marathon runner, but was forced to give it all up after being diagnosed with a rare cardiac condition,

ARVC. She is the author of *Racing Heart: A Runner's Journey of Love, Loss and Perseverance.*

Contact: kate@precisionpt.org
Website: www.precisionpt.org

Dr. Blair Green PT, DPT, is a certified pelvic health practitioner (PHC) and a board-certified orthopaedic clinical specialist (OCS). She is the founder and CEO of Catalyst Physical Therapy in Atlanta, Georgia. She is a faculty member of Evidence in Motion Institute for Health Professions and Myopain Seminars, providing continuing education to physical therapists who are pursuing knowledge of pelvic health.

She also is a guest lecturer for Emory University School of Medicine in the department of physical therapy, teaching doctoral students about pregnancy and pelvic health. She has written for various publications and is a contributing author to *Trigger Point Dry Needling: An Evidence and Clinical-Based Approach*, 2nd edition. Her clinical interests include serving pre- and postnatal women, as well as females across their entire lifespan. A mom of two, her own pregnancy/childbirth experiences and recovery play an important role in her approach to patient care and her desire to establish postnatal physical therapy screening as a standard of care for all women.

Contact: blair@catalystga.com
Website: www.catalystga.com

References

1. Tenforde AS, Toth KE, Langen E, Fredericson M, Sainani KL. Running habits of competitive runners during pregnancy and breastfeeding. *Sports Health*. 2015;7(2):172-176.

2. Yamato TP, Saragiotto BT, Lopes AD. A consensus definition of running-related injury in recreational runners: a modified Delphi approach. *J Orthop Sports Phys Ther*. 2015;45(5):375-380.

3. van der Worp MP, ten Haaf DS, van Cingel R, de Wijer A, Nijhuis-van der Sanden MW, Staal JB. Injuries in runners; a systematic review on risk factors and sex differences. *PLoS One*. 2015;10(2):e0114937.

4. van Gent RN, Siem D, van Middelkoop M, van Os AG, Bierma-Zeinstra SM, Koes BW. Incidence and determinants of lower extremity running injuries in long distance runners: a systematic review. *Br J Sports Med*. 2007;41(8):469-480; discussion 480.

5. Davis IS, Futrell E. Gait Retraining: Altering the Fingerprint of Gait. *Phys Med Rehabil Clin N Am*. 2016;27(1):339-355.

6. Werner W.K. Hoeger LB, Lynda Ransdell, Jane M. Shimon, Sunitha Merugu. One-mile Step Count at Walking and Running Speeds. *ACSM's HEALTH & FITNESS JOURNAL*. 2008;12(1).

7.   Hreljac A. Impact and Overuse Injuries in Runners. *Medicine & Science in Sports & Exercise.* 2004:845-849.

8.   Napier C, Esculier JF, Hunt MA. Gait retraining: out of the lab and onto the streets with the benefit of wearables. *Br J Sports Med.* 2017;51(23):1642-1643.

9.   Napier C, Cochrane CK, Taunton JE, Hunt MA. Gait modifications to change lower extremity gait biomechanics in runners: a systematic review. *Br J Sports Med.* 2015;49(21):1382-1388.

10.   Lynch SL, Hoch AZ. The female runner: gender specifics. *Clin Sports Med.* 2010;29(3):477-498.

11.   Bahr R. No injuries, but plenty of pain? On the methodology for recording overuse symptoms in sports. *Br J Sports Med.* 2009;43(13):966-972.

12.   Messier SP, Martin DF, Mihalko SL, et al. A 2-Year Prospective Cohort Study of Overuse Running Injuries: The Runners and Injury Longitudinal Study (TRAILS). *Am J Sports Med.* 2018;46(9):2211-2221.

13.   Saragiotto BT, Yamato TP, Hespanhol Junior LC, Rainbow MJ, Davis IS, Lopes AD. What are the main risk factors for running-related injuries? *Sports Med.* 2014;44(8):1153-1163.

14.   Hreljac A. Etiology, prevention, and early intervention of overuse injuries in runners: a biomechanical perspective. *Phys Med Rehabil Clin N Am.* 2005;16(3):651-667, vi.

15.   Thein-Nissenbaum J. The postpartum triathlete. *Phys Ther Sport.* 2016;21:95-106.

16.   Charkoudian N, Joyner MJ. Physiologic considerations for exercise performance in women. *Clin Chest Med.* 2004;25(2):247-255.

17.   Kuwahara T, Inoue Y, Abe M, Sato Y, Kondo N. Effects of menstrual cycle and physical training on heat loss responses during dynamic exercise at moderate intensity in a temperate environment. *Am J Physiol Regul Integr Comp Physiol.* 2005;288(5):R1347-1353.

18.   Ichinose TK, Inoue Y, Hirata M, Shamsuddin AK, Kondo

N. Enhanced heat loss responses induced by short-term endurance training in exercising women. *Exp Physiol.* 2009;94(1):90-102.

19. Kim BY, Nattiv A. Health Considerations in Female Runners. *Phys Med Rehabil Clin N Am.* 2016;27(1):151-178.

20. Ireland ML. Hip Strength in Females With and Without Patellofemoral Pain. *JOSPT.* 2003;33(11):671-676.

21. Ferber R, Hreljac A, Kendall KD. Suspected mechanisms in the cause of overuse running injuries: a clinical review. *Sports Health.* 2009;1(3):242-246.

22. Souza RB. An Evidence-Based Videotaped Running Biomechanics Analysis. *Phys Med Rehabil Clin N Am.* 2016;27(1):217-236.

23. FAQ ACOG pregnancy exercise guidelines. *American College of Obstetricians and Gynecologists.* 2017.

24. Bo K, Artal R, Barakat R, et al. Exercise and pregnancy in recreational and elite athletes: 2016 evidence summary from the IOC expert group meeting, Lausanne. Part 2-the effect of exercise on the fetus, labour and birth. *Br J Sports Med.* 2016.

25. Medicine Io. Weight Gain in Pregnancy. *Institute of Medicine.* 2009:1-4.

26. Wanda Forckek RS. Changes of kinematic gait parameters due to pregnancy. *Acta of Bioengineering and Biomechanics.* 2012;14(4):113-119.

27. Stephenson RG OCL. *Obstetric and Gynecologic Care in Physical Therapy.* 2nd ed. Thorofare, NJ: SLACK, Incorporated; 2000.

28. Reese ME, Casey E. Hormonal Influence on the Neuromusculoskeletal System in Pregnancy. In: C.M. Fitzgerald NASe, ed. *Musculoskeletal Health in Pregnancy and Postpartum.* Switzerland: Springer International Publishing 2015:19-39.

29. Clapp J. *Exercising Through Your Pregnancy.* 1st ed. Omaha, NE: Addicus Books; 2002.

30. Lee DG, Hodges, PW. Behavior of the Linea Alba During a Curl-up Task in Diastasis Rectus Abdominis: An Observational Study. *J Orthop Sports Phys Ther.* 2016;46(7):580-589.

31. Keiko L. Torgersen, Curran CA. A Systematic Approach to the Physiologic Adaptations of Pregnancy. *Crit Care Nursing Q.* 2006;29(1):2-19.

32. Carpes FP GD, Kleinpaul JF, Mann L, Mota CB. Women able-bodied gait kinematics during and post pregnancy period. *Brazilian Journal of Biomechanics.* 2008;9(16):34-39.

33. Gilleard WL. Trunk motion and gait characteristics of pregnant women when walking: report of a longitudinal study with a control group. *BMC Pregnancy and Childbirth.* 2013;3(71):1-8.

34. Opinion C. ACOG Post Natal Care Committee Opinion. *Obstetricians and Gynecologists.* 2018;131(5):140-150.

35. Hartmann D, Sarton J. Chronic pelvic floor dysfunction. *Best Pract Res Clin Obstet Gynaecol.* 2014;28(7):977-990.

36. Sapsford RR, Hodges PW. The effect of abdominal and pelvic floor muscle activation on urine flow in women. *Int Urogynecol J.* 2012;23(9):1225-1230.

37. Lee D. The One-Leg Standing Test and the Active Straight Leg Raise Test: A Clinical Interpretation of Two Tests of Load Transfer through the Pelvic Girdle. *Orthopedic Division Review.* 2005.

38. Hans Peter Dietz VL. Levator Trauma After Vaginal Delivery. *OBSTETRICS & GYNECOLOGY.* 2005;106(4):707-712.

39. A. Wong C. Incidence of postpartum lumbosacral spine and lower extremity nerve injuries. *Obstetrics & Gynecology.* 2003;101(2):279-288.

40. Dunbar A, Ernst A, Matthews C, Ramakrishnan V. Understanding Vaginal Childbirth. *Journal of Women's Health Physical Therapy.* 2011;35(2):51-56.

41. Colleran HL, Wideman L, Lovelady CA. Effects of energy

restriction and exercise on bone mineral density during lactation. *Med Sci Sports Exerc.* 2012;44(8):1570-1579.

42. Lovelady CA, Bopp MJ, Colleran HL, Mackie HK, Wideman L. Effect of exercise training on loss of bone mineral density during lactation. *Med Sci Sports Exerc.* 2009;41(10):1902-1907.

43. Krebs NF RC, Robertson AD, Brenner M. Bone mineral density changes during lactation: maternal, dietary, and biomechanical correlates. *Am J Clin Nutr.* 1997;65:1738-1746.

44. Kalkwarf HJ. Changes in Bone Density During Lactation and Weaning. *J Mammary Gland Biol Neoplasia.* 1999;4(3):319-329.

45. Speziali A, Tei MM, Placella G, Chillemi M, Cerulli G. Postpartum Sacral Stress Fracture: An Atypical Case Report. *Case Rep Orthop.* 2015;2015:704393.

46. Tenforde AS, Kraus E, Fredericson M. Bone Stress Injuries in Runners. *Phys Med Rehabil Clin N Am.* 2016;27(1):139-149.

47. Dewey KG. Energy During Lactation. *Annual Review Nutrition.* 1997(17):19-36.

48. Butte NF, King JC. Energy requirements during pregnancy and lactation. *Public Health Nutrition.* 2007;8(7a).

49. Iwata H, Mori E, Sakajo A, Aoki K, Maehara K, Tamakoshi K. Course of maternal fatigue and its associated factors during the first 6 months postpartum: a prospective cohort study. *Nurs Open.* 2018;5(2):186-196.

50. Palazzetti S, Margaritis I, Guezennec CY. Swimming and cycling overloaded training in triathlon has no effect on running kinematics and economy. *Int J Sports Med.* 2005;26(3):193-199.

51. Svabik K, Shek KL, Dietz HP. How much does the levator hiatus have to stretch during childbirth? *BJOG.* 2009;116(12):1657-1662.

52. Dufour S, Vandyken B, Forget MJ, Vandyken C. Association between lumbopelvic pain and pelvic floor dysfunction in women: A cross sectional study. *Musculoskelet Sci Pract.*

2018;34:47-53.

53.   Clifton S, Tania, Rowley J. Breathing pattern disorders
       and physiotherapy: inspiration for our profession. *Physical
       Therapy Reviews.* 2013;16(1):75-86.

54.   Michelle D Smith AR, Paul Hodges. Disorders of breathing
       and continence have a stronger association with back pain
       than obesity and physical activity. *Australian Journal of
       Physiotherapy.* 2006;52.

55.   Michelle D Smith AR, Paul Hodges. The Relationship
       Between Incontinence, Breathing Disorders, Gastrointestinal
       Symptoms, and Back Pain in Women. *Clinical Journal of Pain.*
       2013;00(00):1-6.

56.   Britt Stuge EL, Gitle Kirkesola, and Nina Vøllestad. The
       Efficacy of a Treatment Program Focusing on Specific
       Stabilizing Exercises for Pelvic Girdle Pain After Pregnancy:
       A Randomized Controlled Trial. *Spine.* 2004;29(4):351-359.

57.   Abrams P, Cardozo L, Fall M, et al. The standardisation of
       terminology of lower urinary tract function: report from
       the Standardisation Sub-committee of the International
       Continence Society. *Neurourol Urodyn.* 2002;21(2):167-178.

58.   Boyle R H-SE, Cody JD, Mørkved S. Pelvic floor muscle
       training for prevention and treatment of urinary and faecal
       incontinence in antenatal and postnatal women (Review).
       The Cochrane Library. 2012(10):1112.

59.   Ashton-Miller JA, Delancey JOL. Functional Anatomy of
       the Female Pelvic Floor. *Annals of the New York Academy of
       Sciences.* 2007;1101(1):266-296.

60.   Hagen S, Stark D, Glazener C, et al. Individualised pelvic
       floor muscle training in women with pelvic organ prolapse
       (POPPY): a multicentre randomised controlled trial. *The
       Lancet.* 2014;383(9919):796-806.

61.   Hagen S SD. Conservative prevention and management of
       pelvic organ prolapse in women (Review). *The Cochrane
       Library.* 2011(12).

62.   Vleeming A, Albert HB, Ostgaard HC, Sturesson B, Stuge

B. European guidelines for the diagnosis and treatment of pelvic girdle pain. *Eur Spine J.* 2008;17(6):794-819.

63. Spitznagle TM, Leong FC, Van Dillen LR. Prevalence of diastasis recti abdominis in a urogynecological patient population. *Int Urogynecol J Pelvic Floor Dysfunct.* 2007;18(3):321-328.

64. Petersen J, Sorensen H, Nielsen RO. Cumulative loads increase at the knee joint with slow-speed running compared to faster running: a biomechanical study. *J Orthop Sports Phys Ther.* 2015;45(4):316-322.

65. Borg-Stein J, Dugan SA, Gruber J. Musculoskeletal Aspects of Pregnancy. *American Journal of Physical Medicine & Rehabilitation.* 2005;84(3):180-192.

66. Pivarnik J. Impact of physical activity during pregnancy and postpartum on chronic disease risk. *Med Sci Sports Exerc.* 2006;38(5):989-1006.

67. Brembeck P, Lorentzon M, Ohlsson C, Winkvist A, Augustin H. Changes in cortical volumetric bone mineral density and thickness, and trabecular thickness in lactating women postpartum. *J Clin Endocrinol Metab.* 2015;100(2):535-543.

68. Brooks AaD, Benjamin. Acetabular Labral tear and Postpartum Hip Pain. *Obstetricians and Gynecologists.* 2012;120(5).

69. Thein-Nissenbaum JM, Thompson EF, Chumanov ES, Heiderscheit BC. Low back and hip pain in a postpartum runner: applying ultrasound imaging and running analysis. *J Orthop Sports Phys Ther.* 2012;42(7):615-624.

70. Rathleff MS, Molgaard CM, Fredberg U, et al. High-load strength training improves outcome in patients with plantar fasciitis: A randomized controlled trial with 12-month follow-up. *Scand J Med Sci Sports.* 2015;25(3):e292-300.

71. Heiderscheit B. The Runner: Evaluation of Common Injuries and Treatment. In: Hoffman CHS, ed. *Orthopeadic Management of the Runner, Cyclist, and Swimmer (Section 1).* 1st ed: APTA 2013.

72. Van Leeuwen KDB. RJ, Winzenberg T., van Middlekoop M. Higher body mass index is associated with plantar fasciopathy/'plantar fasciitis': systematic review and meta-analysis of various clinical and imaging risk factors. *Br J Sports Med* 2016;50(16):972-981.

73. Lee DG, Lee LJ, McLaughlin L. Stability, continence and breathing: the role of fascia following pregnancy and delivery. *J Bodyw Mov Ther.* 2008;12(4):333-348.

74. Nguyen John LL, Choe Jennifer, McKindsey Francis, Sinow Robert, Bhatia Narender Lumbosacral spine and pelvic inlet changes associated with pelvic organ prolapse. *Obstetrics & Gynecology.* 2000;5(3):332-336.

75. Bo K, Artal R, Barakat R, et al. Exercise and pregnancy in recreational and elite athletes: 2016 evidence summary from the IOC expert group meeting, Lausanne. Part 1-exercise in women planning pregnancy and those who are pregnant. *Br J Sports Med.* 2016;50(10):571-589.

76. Pappas PT, Paradisis GP, Exell TA, Smirniotou AS, Tsolakis CK, Arampatzis A. Acute Effects of Stretching on Leg and Vertical Stiffness During Treadmill Running. *J Strength Cond Res.* 2017;31(12):3417-3424.

77. Fletcher I. The effect of different dynamic stretch velocities on jump performance. *Eur J Appl Physiol* 2010(109):491-498.

78. O'Sullivan R, Kiernan D, Malone A. Run kinematics with and without a jogging stroller. *Gait Posture.* 2016;43:220-224.

79. Gregory DA, Pfeiffer KA, Vickers KE, et al. Physiologic responses to running with a jogging stroller. *Int J Sports Med.* 2012;33(9):711-715.

80. G.A. Brown MPR, M.L. Scott, J. Harris III, M.K. Colaluca, B.S. Shaw and I. Shaw. Physiological and biomechanical responses of running with and without a stroller : sport and physical activity. *African Journal for Physical Health Education, Recreation and Dance.* 2008;14(3):240-249.